Laparoscopic Techniques in Small Animal Surgery

About the Authors

Dr Swapan Kumar Maiti, a graduate from Bidhan Chandra Krishi Viswa Vidyalaya (1984) followed by Masters (1987) and Doctorate (1990) in Veterinary Surgery from Indian Veterinary Research Institute. Dr Maiti joined ICAR-Indian Veterinary Research Institute as Scientist in 1993 and currently working as Principal Scientist in this Premier Indian Institute. Presently, Dr Maiti has more than 25 years of research experience in the field of Animal Oncology, Laparoscopic Surgery and Animal Stem Cells Biology.

He is associated with more than 20 research projects and published more than 200 research and clinical papers in different peer reviewed International and National journals and presented more than 100 scientific papers in International and National Congress. Besides, he has authored two Text-books, three manuals, two compendiums and contributed twenty chapters in different books.

Dr Maiti has been invited as "Speaker" in the 32nd, 33rd, 35th, 36th and 38th World Small Animal Veterinary Association (WSAVA) World Congress, held at Sydney (Australia); Dublin (Ireland); Geneva (Switzerland), Jeju (South Korea) and Auckland (New Zealand) respectively. He has also been invited as "Speaker" in the 2nd Federation of Asian Small Animal Veterinary Association (FASAVA) Congress held at Bangkok (Thailand) in 2009. So far, he has visited more than 25 countries on different scientific assignments.

He has been awarded prestigious fellowship from German Research Foundation (DFG), Germany for Post-Doctoral research work under International Bilateral Scientist Exchange Programme of Govt. of India. Dr Maiti deputed as "Visiting Professor" at the University of Leipzig (2006), University of Köln (2010) and Technical University of Munich (2014), Germany.

He has guided eight M.V.Sc, one M. Pharm and seven Ph.D students. He received many prestigious awards in his academic career including Prof A.K. Bhargava Gold Medal, Shri Ramlal Agrawal National Award (Gold Medal & Cash Prize); Prof S.J. Angelo Memorial Award, Indian Science Congress Centenary Best Paper (Certificate and Cash prize) and also nominated as "International Expert" for assessment of teachers of Foreign University (Sudan) for three years. Dr Maiti is a "Fellow" of National Academy of Veterinary Sciences, Indian Society for Veterinary Surgery and Indian Society for Advancement of Canine Practice for outstanding contribution in the field of Veterinary Science.

Dr Naveen Kumar is working as Principal Scientist in the Division of Surgery, ICAR-Indian Veterinary Research Institute, Izatnagar. He has rich blend of teaching and research experience in the field of Veterinary Surgery for more than 28 years. During his illustrious career he has been associated in 15 Research projects of which 5 were externally funded projects. He has done pioneering research work in the area of Veterinary Surgery especially in the field of biomaterials. He developed concept for development of biomaterials from abattoir waste for reconstructive surgery for the first time in India. A new concept of application of laparoscopy in clinical diagnosis and therapeutics in veterinary patients was developed by him. He has also filed one patent for the process development of biomaterials and published more than 300 Research papers in International and National Journals of repute having high impact factors.

In recognition of significant contributions for the advancement of Veterinary Sciences, Dr Kumar has been elected Fellow of National Academy of Veterinary Sciences. His research work has fetched him several awards including Ramani Ramchandran Award, Gangman Sharma Award, Best oral presentation award from Indian Society for Veterinary Surgery and Indian Society for Veterinary Medicine and several Appreciation Awards. Dr Kumar has written 6 Books, 5 Manuals and more than 40 chapters in Books and Manuals in the field of Surgery. He has presented more than 200 papers in National and International Conferences and guided 10 M.V.Sc. and 4 Ph.D. students. He has delivered more than 30 lectures as Invited Speaker in different conferences and forums.

A Colour Book
Laparoscopic Techniques in Small Animal Surgery

Swapan Kumar Maiti
Naveen Kumar

NEW INDIA PUBLISHING AGENCY
New Delhi – 110 034

NEW INDIA PUBLISHING AGENCY
101, Vikas Surya Plaza, CU Block, LSC Market
Pitam Pura, New Delhi 110 034, India
Phone: + 91 (11)27 34 17 17 Fax: + 91(11) 27 34 16 16
Email: info@nipabooks.com
Web: www.nipabooks.com

Feedback at feedbacks@nipabooks.com

ISBN 978-93-85516-56-6

Composed and Designed by NIPA.

Acknowledgement

We are thankful to the Indian Council of Agricultural Research, New Delhi for approving and funding one research project on laparoscopic studies in animals, which is the base for this publication. We are grateful to the Director, Indian Veterinary Research Institute, Izatnagar (UP) and Head, Surgery Division, IVRI, Izatnagar for their generous help and support towards this publication. Thanks are also due to all the scientific, technical and supporting staff of the Surgery Division, IVRI without their help it would not have been possible to complete this task. We wish to acknowledge the authors and publishers of different reference books/papers consulted for the preparation of this task. Help and wholehearted support extended by the learned faculty members in general and some PG students of Surgery Division, IVRI especially Drs Avijit Dutta, Ajith P, Anbu Raja, Ninu A R, Mathew D, Dileep Kumar, Tamil Mahan, Sangeetha P and Divya Mohan in particular to bring out the publication are duly acknowledged.

Inspiration, suggestion and personal helps by Prof. (Dr) David C. Twedt, Internationally reputed laparoscopic surgeon and Diplomate ACVIM, Department of Clinical Sciences, College of Veterinary Medicine and Biomedical Science, Colorado State University, Fort Collins, USA is highly acknowledged.

Last, but not the least our special heartiest thanks and sincere appreciation to our family for their patience, devotion, deep understanding and cooperation to accomplish this arduous task.

We would appreciate to receive any suggestion and constructive criticism about the publication and our efforts would be to further improve more subject and latest information in the next edition.

Hope our efforts would help to propagate this minimally invasive techniques to the veterinary clinicians and students in alleviates the suffering of pain in animals.

Dated: IVRI, Izatnagar
17th February, 2016

Swapan Kumar Maiti
Naveen Kumar

Contents

List of Colour Plates

1

Introduction

Laparoscope

The term laparoscope derived from Greek word "Laparo" meaning "flank," which is the side of the body between the ribs and hips (abdomen) and "scope" means to look at or examine. Laparoscope can be defined as an instrument through which structures within the abdomen and pelvis can be seen or a *fiber optic* device that consists of a flexible tube. Fiber optic scope is used to directly visualize the internal anatomy of a hollow organ. Laparoscope is used in *laparoscopy* and *laparoscopic* surgery. It has lenses like a telescope to magnify body structures, a powerful light to illuminate them and a miniature video camera. The camera sends images of the inside of the body to a TV monitor in the operating room. Specialized surgical instruments can be inserted through the laparoscope.

Laparoscopy

Laparoscopy (pronounced "lap-a-ROSS-coe-pee") is a surgical procedure performed through very small incisions in the abdomen, using specialized instruments. A pencil-thin instrument called a laparoscope is used, and it gives the surgeon an exceptionally clear view on a TV monitor of the inside of the abdominal cavity. Laparoscopy is an endoscopic procedure designed for the visual examination and biopsy of the peritoneal cavity and its organs. It is used to examine the interior of the abdominal or pelvic cavities for the diagnosis or treatment (or both) of number of diseases and conditions. Laparoscopy is a surgical procedure in which a small incision is made, usually in the abdomen, through which a viewing tube (laparoscope) is inserted. The viewing tube has a small camera on the eyepiece. This allows the surgeon to examine the abdominal and pelvic organs on a video monitor connected to the tube. Other small incisions can be made to insert accessory instruments to perform different surgical procedures including biopsy collection from different abdominal organs.

This type of surgery is called 'minimally invasive' because of the very small incisions used. Yet major procedures can now be performed using this technique. The term laparoscopy is used when this type of surgery is performed in the abdomen. It's called arthroscopy when performed in a joint and endoscopy when done through a natural opening in the body, such as the mouth or nose. The advantage of laparoscopy is that only a small incision (minimally invasive technique) is required; this is why laparoscopy is also known as 'Keyhole surgery'.

Fundamentals of minimally invasive surgery (MIS)

Laparoscopic techniques have become important in veterinary medicine in the last 10 years. In human medicine, laparoscopy has become the gold standard of many abdominal procedures. MIS in humans has been shown to have numerous advantages over traditional celiotomy/ laparotomy techniques including: improved visualization of abdominal organs, shorter postoperative stress and pain, faster recovery periods, decreased hospital stays, improved cosmetic and early rehabilitation. However, some veterinary surgeons have avoided this modality due to inherent limitations of minimally invasive surgery, including cost of equipment, procedural learning curve and increased time of the procedure compared to traditional surgical techniques.

Laparoscopy is a minimally invasive technique for directly viewing the internal structures of the abdominal cavity. Direct visualization of the organ helps the clinician to imply an assiduous control and accurate site localization of the various organs. The invasiveness of the procedure, rapid patient recovery and diagnostic accuracy make laparoscopy ideal techniques over many other invasive procedures. Small animal laparoscopy has not only developed into a diagnostic tool but more recently has progressed to where it has become a means for minimally invasive surgical procedures.

The equipment required for laparoscopy consists of a laparoscope, light source, insufflator and video imaging capabilities. Laparoscopes are available in a variety of sizes ranging from 2.7mm to 10mm and angles ranging from 0 to 70 degrees. The angled telescopes give the ability to see around corners, especially when working in a compact area. It is common in veterinary medicine to use a 10mm scope with a 30degree angle. Light is transmitted to the telescope via fiber optic cable from a remote light source. Xenon (300watt) and halogen (150watt) are the most commonly used light sources. The magnification of the telescope and light source allows the surgeon to see details and pathology not observable to the naked eye.

Insufflation is performed using carbon dioxide, nitrous oxide, or room air. Air is insufflated into the abdominal cavity via a Veress needle. Abdominal pressure should be insufflated to 10-12 mmHg. Pressure higher than 15mmHg can result in decreased venous return to the heart and impair ventilation. A complication of laparoscopic surgery is the possibility of air embolism. Carbon dioxide is the preferred gas for insufflation due to its high solubility and rapid absorption. The risk for emboli increases when insufflation occurs in a hollow viscous and when room air is used, due to its poor solubility.

Video capabilities are directed around the camera and its video output system. Charge-coupled semiconductor cameras, also called "chip cameras", have differing levels of resolution based upon the number of chips provided internally. Three-chip cameras operate with 1 chip for each of the primary colors and have the best resolution. Cameras with high-resolution output require less light source for image detail. Video capture systems can allow for procedural documentation of pathology, photos, and facilitates teaching. Most laparoscopic equipment setups place the video tower in direct view of the camera operator to reduce operator fatigue in surgery.

In humans it has been well documented that laparoscopic surgery results in less pain and morbidity, as well as, shorter hospital stays when compared to open surgical techniques. Laparoscopic surgery is less painful due to smaller incision size, decreased muscular trauma and earlier return to function. Using canine models to perfect human techniques limited published veterinary reports have described the feasibility, safety, and efficacy of laparoscopic surgery for gastropexy, ovariohysterectomy, nephrectomy, proximal gastric vagotomy, cholecystectomy, prostatectomy, cryptorchidectomy, small intestinal anastomosis and colectomy.

Uses of laparoscopy

Laparoscopy can be done to diagnose conditions or to perform certain types of operations. It is less invasive than regular open abdominal surgery (laparotomy). Prior to the advent of laparoscopy, doctors had to make large openings and cut through layers of tissue in order to examine internal organs. Laparoscopy greatly reduces the patient's recovery time. Laparoscopy is simple to perform and considered to be safe having very few complications. Despite the advent of newer laboratory tests, imaging techniques and ultrasound directed fine needle biopsy or aspiration; laparoscopy remains a valuable tool when appropriately applied in a diagnostic plan.

Laparoscopy can be used in the following procedures:

- The *diagnosis* of the disease conditions
  - By biopsy i.e. histopathology
  - By direct visualization of the body cavity through laparoscope
- The surgical *treatment* of the diseases
- *Biopsy* of the abdominal organs or masses
- The *examination* of the different body cavity organs

Diagnostic laparoscopy

Diagnostic laparoscopy is a procedure that allows looking directly at the contents of a patient's abdomen or pelvis, including the fallopian tubes, ovaries, uterus, small bowel, large bowel, appendix, liver, and gallbladder. Diagnostic laparoscopy is indicated when inspection of the abdomen will establish a diagnosis and to define subsequent treatment. Diagnostic laparoscopy is commonly used as a method for obtaining liver, pancreas, and kidney, splenic and intestinal biopsies. It is generally accepted that laparoscopy provides better liver biopsy tissues than other traditional percutaneous methods. Laparoscopy is also used in oncology to diagnose and stage the extent of malignancy; either primary or metastatic. Unexplained abdominal effusion is an additional indication for performing the procedure when other diagnostics are unsuccessful. Patients that are to undergo endoscopic surgery should have a complete preoperative evaluation prior to scheduling the surgery. The preoperative evaluation often includes laboratory and echographic examination in order to determine the clear indication for surgery.

Indication for diagnostic laparoscopy

- *Infertility*: This is one of the most common indications for diagnostic laparoscopy. The conditions which can be diagnosed by laparoscopy include:
  - Adhesions- evidence of prior pelvic infection.
  - Structural abnormalities of the uterus, including congenital developmental abnormalities (such as a bicornuate or unicornuate uterus) and fibroids.
  - Endometritis.
- *Chronic abdominal pain*: The systematic evaluation of the abdomen and pelvis provided key diagnostic information in the evaluation of an animal with chronic pelvic pain. In particular, the laparoscopy may reveal adhesions or endometriosis not visible by other diagnostic techniques.
- *Ectopic Pregnancy*: Laparoscopy for ectopic pregnancy often not only provides the diagnosis but also allows for the immediate surgical treatment.
- *Liver biopsy*
- *Pancreatic biopsy*
- *Kidney biopsy*
- *Intestinal biopsy*
- *Cholecystocentesis*
- *Adrenal evaluation*
- *Splenic evaluation*
- *Reproductive evaluation*
- *Diseases of the urinary system*: Laparoscopy can be used to investigate or treat (or both) cancerous and non-cancerous conditions of the kidney, blockages of the ureter, bladder disease and incontinence.

- *Cancers of the internal organs*: Cancers of the liver and pancreas can be diagnosed using laparoscopy.
- *Ascites*: Laparoscopy can help determine the cause.
- *Abdominal cryptorchidism*

Indication for surgical laparoscopy

- *Enterostomy/gastrostomy feeding tube placement*
- *Repair of rectal and colonic tear*
- *Tube cystotomy in urolitheasis*
- *Gastropexy*
- *Ovariohysterectomy*
- *Bilateral oophorectomy*
- *Cryptorchid surgery*
- *Gastric foreign body removal*
- *Cystoscopy*
- *Vasectomy*
- *Vasectomy and endoclipping of spermatic plexus*

Examination of the organs of body cavity

Laparoscope is also used for the examinations of the organs of the body cavity for their anatomy, whether it is normal or abnormal. Simultaneous diagnosis can be done if it is found abnormal. Liver, gall bladder, stomach, abdominal esophagus, small and large intestine, spleen, kidney etc. are examined for their shape, size, location, color and even consistency. During the examination the different disease conditions which can be diagnosed are hepatomegaly, spleenomegaly, torsion and volvulus of the stomach and intestine, abnormal body fluid i.e. ascites etc.

Advantages and Disadvantages

Laparoscopy is a unique surgical approach that shares characteristics of both minor and major surgery. To patients, laparoscopic procedures are often considered minor surgery because of the small incisions, relatively small amount of postoperative pain, and short convalescent period. The advantages of surgical laparoscopy over the conventional open surgical laparotomy include improved patient recovery because of smaller surgical incision, lower postoperative morbidity with less infection rate and postoperative pain. Another advantage of laparoscopy is less surgical stress. Physiologic responses that account for improved clinical outcome with laparoscopy have been studied extensively and find less impairment of metabolism, renal and pulmonary workload with better bowel motility and immune function when compared to similar open surgical procedures performing similar manipulations.

At its essence, laparoscopy remains an intra-abdominal procedure. Therefore, it shares all intraoperative and postoperative risks of laparotomy, including infection and injury to adjacent intra-abdominal structures. When major intra-abdominal procedures are performed laparoscopically (e.g. hysterectomy), the resultant postoperative pain and morbidity are still significant. However, because a large abdominal incision is unnecessary, the postoperative pain and morbidity are always less significant than similar major surgery performed by routine laparotomy.

Laparoscopic procedures have unique risks, which are related to methods used for the placement of abdominal wall ports and to the pneumoperitoneum required for laparoscopy. These risks include injury to bowel, bladder or major blood vessels and intravascular insufflation. In addition, increased intra-abdominal pressures associated with laparoscopy increases anesthesia related risks such as aspiration and increased difficulty in ventilating the patient. Although the risk of blood loss is relatively low for most procedures, potentially massive blood loss may occur and is complicated by the fact that control of blood loss may be delayed by the time taken to perform an emergency laparotomy. The downside of surgical laparoscopy is the cost of some of the specialized surgical instruments and stapling and electrocautery devices.

Contraindications

Laparoscopy and organ biopsy should not be performed in animals with coagulopathy. Extensive intra abdominal adhesions from previous surgery or disease can result in visceral puncture during laparoscopy; therefore exploratory laparotomy is recommended in these individuals. Profound ascites can complicate laparoscopy and increases the likelihood of visceral puncture. Bacterial or septic peritonitis and abdominal herniation (diaphragmatic or inguinal) are obvious contraindications. Other relative contraindications include the patient condition, small body size or obesity. The procedure becomes difficult in the very small patient (less than 2 kg b wt) as reduce working space. Animals having excessive intra-abdominal body fat often obscure the view of many organs thus making the procedure much more difficult to perform.

Complications

Giving attention to proper technique can minimize complications during and after laparoscopy. The following complications can occur during or after laparoscopy.

- Puncture of hollow organs (stomach, urinary bladder or intestine) during establishment of pneumoperitoneum resulting in gas distention of organs.
- Puncture of abdominal wall vascular.
- Penetration of organs.
- Anesthesia related.
- Occurrence of gas embolism after placement of Veress needle placement.
- Subcutaneous emphysema due to improper Veress needle placement.
- Peritoneal tenting.
- Pneumothorax.
- Operative complications.
- Cardiopulmonary compromise due to excessive pneumoperitoneum.
- Trocar punctures of visceral organs due to faulty technique.
- Inadvertent puncture of vessels or structures due to biopsy needle.

- Excessive hemorrhage from the biopsy site.
- Equipment related problems.
- Bile peritonitis.
- Bacterial peritonitis.
- Electro caution.

❑❑❑

2

History

The early history of laparoscopy is unknown to many surgeons, but Hippocrates (460-375 BC) in Greece was first to describe endoscopy). He made reference to a rectal speculum. Hippocrates also advised injecting a large quantity of air into the intestines through the anus in the case of intestinal obstruction. He also advocated the insertion of suppository that was 10 digits long. These descriptions suggest that Hippocrates was well aware of ileus with intestinal obstruction and thought of several possible etiologies, including faecal impaction, intussusception, and sigmoid volvulus. Moreover, Hippocrates treated these life-threatening conditions with minimally invasive approaches.

The first simple speculum for gynecological endoscopy dates from about the same time. Roman medicine also produced instruments with which they could inspect internal organs. In Pompeii's ruins (70 AD), a three-bladed vaginal speculum was found; this instrument was similar to the modern vaginal speculum. Albukasim, an Arab doctor of the 11th century, developed a speculum illuminated by a set of light reflectors. Thus the interest for physicians to look into the "internal organs" has existed since the early days of medicine.

The history of laparoscopy/endoscopy in chronological order is mentioned bellow:

1585 : Aranzi was the first to use a light source for an endoscopic procedure, focusing sunlight through a flask of water and projecting the light into the nasal cavity.

1706 : The term "trocar" was coined in 1706 and was thought to be derived from trochartor troise-quarts, a three-faced instrument consisting of a perforator enclosed in a metal cannula.

1806 : Philip Bozzini (1773-1809) built an instrument that could be introduced in the human body to visualize the internal organs. He called this instrument "LICHTLEITER". Bozzini used an aluminium tube to visualize the genitourinary tract. The tube, illuminated by a wax candle, had fitted mirrors to reflect image. Bozzini's invention established the principles that guided the development of endoscopy and it inspired others to forge ahead in this new fields.

1840 : John D. Fisher (1798-1850) in Boston described an endoscope initially to inspect the vagina, but later he modified it to examine the bladder and urethra.

1853 : Antoine Jean Desormeaux, a French surgeon first introduced the 'Lichtleiter" of Bozzini to a patient. For many surgeons he is considered as the "Father of Endoscopy". The Lichtleiter was mainly used for urologic cases. Many developments, which occurred independently but almost simultaneously, produced breakthroughs for endoscopy and laparoscopy that were the bases for modern instruments. In this period the invention of incandescent light was intended.

1860 : Maximilian Nitze (1848-1906) modified Edison's light bulb invention and created the first electrical light bulb as the source of illumination.

1867 : Desormeaux, used an open tube to examine the genitourinary tract, combining alcohol and turpentine with a flame in order to generate a brighter, more condensable beam of light.

1868 : Kussmaul performed the first esophagogastroscopy on a professional sword swallower, initiating efforts at instrumentation of the gastrointestinal tract. Mikulicz and Schindler, however, are credited with the advancement of gastroscopy.

1869 : Commander Pantaleoni used a modified cystoscope to cauterize a hemorrhagic uterine growth. Pantaleoni thus performed the first diagnostic and therapeutic hysteroscopy.

1883 : Newman of Glasgow described a miniaturized version of the incandescent bulb in a cystoscope.

1901 : Dimitri Ott, wore head mirrors to reflect light and augment visualization and used access technique in which a speculum was introduced through an incision in the prior vaginal fornix.

1901 : The first experimental laparoscopy was performed in Berlin, German surgeon Georg Kelling, who used a cystoscope to peer into the abdomen of a dog_after first insufflating it with air. He also used filtered atmospheric air to create a pneumoperitoneum, with the goal of stopping intra-abdominal bleeding (ectopic pregnancy, bleeding ulcers, and pancreatitis) but these studies did not find any response or supporters. Kelling proposed a high-pressure insulation of the abdominal cavity, a technique he called the "Luft-tamponade" or "air-tamponade".

1911 : Bertram M. Bernheim, an assistant surgeon from Johns Hopkins Hospital introduced first laparoscopic surgery to the United States. He named the procedure of minimal access surgery as "organoscopy". The instrument used was a proctoscope of a half inch diameter and ordinary light for illumination was used.

1911 : H.C. Jacobaeus, from Stockolm, coined the term "laparothorakoskopie". Using this procedure on the thorax and abdomen, he introduced the trocar inside the body cavity directly without employing a pneumoperi-toneum. He published his report on laparoscopy and thoracoscopy in humans in Münchener Medizinische Wochenschrift. He also suggested similar techniques to examine body cavities endoscopically. He was the first person who performed laparoscopy on a human.

1918 : O. Goetze, developed an automatic pneumoperitoneum needle characterized for its safe introduction to the peritoneal cavity. The next decade and a half saw an interruption of technological advances and a lack of any substantial development in endoscopy due to World War I.

1920 : Zollikofer of Switzerland discovered the benefit of CO_2 gas to use for insufflation, rather than filtered atmospheric air or nitrogen.

1929 : Kalk, a German physician, introduced the forward oblique (135 degree) view lens systems. He advocated the use of a separate puncture site for pneumoperitoneum.

1929 : Heinz Kalk, a German gastroenterologist developed a 135-degree lens system and a dual trocar approach. He used laparoscopy as a diagnostic method for liver and gallbladder disease.

1934 : John C. Ruddock, an American surgeon described laparoscopy as a good diagnostic method, many times, superior than laparotomy. He used the instrument for diagnostic laparoscopy, which was consisted a built-in forceps with electrocoagulation capacity.

1938 : Janos Veres of Hungary developed a specially designed spring-loaded needle. Interestingly, Veres did not promote the use of his Veress needle for laparoscopy purposes. He used veress needle for the induction of pneumothorax. Veress needle is the most important instrument today to create pneumo-peritoneum. Veress needle consists of an outer cannula with a beveled needlepoint for cutting through tissues. Inside the cannula of veress needle is an inner stylet, which is loaded with a spring that spring moves forward in response to the sudden decrease in pressure encountered upon crossing the abdominal wall and entering the peritoneal cavity.

1939 : Richard W. Telinde, tried to perform an endoscopic procedure by a culdoscopic approach, in the lithotomy position. This method was rapidly abandoned because of the presence of small intestine.

1939 : Heinz Kalk published his experience of 2000 liver biopsies, performed using local anaesthesia without mortality.

1944 : Raoul Palmer of Paris, performed gynaecological examinations using laparoscopy and placing the patients in the Trendelemburg position, so that air could fill the pelvis. He also stressed the importance of continuous intra-abdominal pressure monitoring during a laparoscopic procedure.

Harold H. Hopkins was responsible for the two most important inventions in endoscopy after World War II. One is the rod-lens system and second is fibreoptic.

1960 : Kurt Semm, a German gynaecologist, who invented the automatic insufflators. His experience with this new device was published in 1966. Although not recognized in his own land, on the other side of the Atlantic, both American physicians and instrument makers valued the Semm insufflator for its simple application, clinical value, and safety.

1966 : Kurt Semm introduced an automatic insufflation device capable of monitoring intra abdominal pressure. This reduced the dangers associated with insufflation of the abdomen and allowed safer laparoscopy.

In 1970's, some gynecologists had embraced laparoscopy and thoroughly incorporated this technique into their practice. General surgeons, despite their exposure to laparoscopy remained confined to traditional open surgery.

1971 : Dr. de Kok invented a technique of laparoscopic appendectomy. An account of his first 30 cases was published in 1977.

1978 : Hasson, introduced an alternative method of trocar placement. He proposed a blunt mini-laparotomy, which permits direct visualization of trocar entrance into the peritoneal cavity. A reusable device of similar design to a standard cannula but attached to an olive-shaped sleeve was developed by Hasson. This sleeve would slide up and down the shaft of the cannula and would form an airtight seal at the fascial opening. In addition, a blunt obturator replaced the sharp trocar. This cannula is held in place by the use of stay sutures passed through the fascial edges and attached to the body of the cannula.

1980 : Patrick Steptoe in United Kingdom started to perform laparoscopic procedures.

1982 : First solid-state camera was introduced. This is the start of "video-laparoscopy".

1983 : Semm, a German gynaecologist, performed the first laparoscopic appendicectomy.

1985 : Erich Mühe in Germany performed the first documented laparoscopic cholecystectomy in 1985.

1987 : Phillipe Mouret, has got the credit to perform the first laparoscopic cholecystectomy in Lyons, France using video technique.

1994 : A robotic arm was designed to hold the telescope with the goal of improving safety and reducing the need of skilled camera operator.

1996 : First live telecast of laparoscopic surgery performed remotely via the Internet. (Robotic telesurgery).

2003 : Van Goethem described monopolar versus bipolar electrocoagulation in canine laparoscopic ovariectomy.

2004 : Uta Delling first described hand-assisted laparoscopic ovariohysterectomy technique in mare.

2004 : Dharmaceelan described one technique of laparoscopic sterilization in bitches.

2006 : Avijit Dutta compared three different techniques of laparoscopic sterilization in bitches.

2006 : Ambu Raja described two techniques of laparoscopic sterilization in male dogs.

2006 : Ajith, P described different laparoscopic ancillary procedures in dogs.

❑❑❑

3

Instrumentation

The basic equipment for performing laparoscopy includes the laparoscope and corresponding trocar and cannula, light source, gas insufflator and the Veress needle. Laparoscope applicable for use in the small animals (dog, goat, sheep and lab animals) ranges in diameter from 2.7 to 10 mm in diameter, however, a 5mm diameter telescope is suitable for most cases and 2.7mm may be required for toy breeds of dogs and lab animals. A 0 or 30 degree direction of vision provides the operator with a "normal' field of view and has proven most useful. Authors are using a 5-mm diameter 30-degree field of view telescope for routine diagnostic laparoscopy. The 5-mm diameter is adequate for most all small animal procedures in animals of variable size. The 0-degree designation means that the telescope views the visual field directly in front of the telescope. The most common being a 30-degree telescope, views in a 30 degree down ward direction. The angled telescope enable the operator to look over the top of organs and view in small areas however this angulations also makes the orientation more difficult for the less experienced operator. Angled telescopes are not generally recommended for the beginner or even needed only performing diagnostic laparoscopy. Smaller diameter (< 3.5mm) telescopes have a more limited field of view, transmit less light for illumination and work best only in the very small animals. The larger diameter telescopes are generally not necessary and in fact often become difficult to use in the very small animals. Following insufflations of the abdominal cavity, telescope and instruments can then be placed through the abdominal cavity by a trocar cannula unit. The trocar and cannula size corresponds to the diameter of the laparoscope being used. Trocar tips are either conical or pyramidal. The pyramidal tip is preferred because it facilitates easier abdominal wall penetration. The cannula consists of a hollow channel to accommodate the telescope with a valve, which prevents insufflation loss while removing the trocar or inserting the laparoscope/telescope. Most all cannula also contain a Leur-lock adapter valve for attachment of the CO_2 hose pipe for continued gas insufflations of the abdominal cavity. A wide variety of light source is available. A light source containing a 150 W lamp is sufficient for routine diagnostic laparoscopy. A flexible fibre optic cable is required to transmit light source to the laparoscope. A flexible 6 mm fibreoptic light transmitting cable is generally advocated for dog to provide more light transmission and hence, better internal illumination. A high intensity light source such as xenon or halogen is recommended for laparoscopy. Xenon is considered to give the truest colors of the abdominal organs and is recommended. Video assisted endoscopy is now considered to be the norm in performing laparoscopy. When an endoscopic video camera is attached to the telescope it allows the image to be viewed on a monitor or coloured television. Video assistance is essential when performing surgical laparoscopy. Video guidance makes laparoscopy much easier to learn and perform. The Veress needle is a spring-loaded, blunt-tipped needle used to establish a pneumo/capnoperitoneum. A Veress needle of 120mm length and equipped with an on-off Luer-lock adapter is suitable for use. The needle consists of an outer sharp cutting tip but contained within the needle is a spring-loaded obturator that retracts into the needle penetrates the abdominal wall. With the internal obturator in place, it prevents needle injury to internal abdominal organs. The hub of the needle is then attached to insufflations tubing that has attached to the automatic gas insufflators. Automatic gas (CO_2) insufflator provides a great deal of convenience and safety during laparoscopic examination by allowing measurement of total gas volume delivered as well as intra-abdominal pressure. Most automatic insufflators are similar in function to deliver gas at a prescribed rate while maintaining a predetermined intra-abdominal pressure. Carbon dioxide is considered to be the gas of choice for insufflations because of the safety factors in preventing air emboli and spark ignition during cauterization. Other equipments and instruments used are standard ones.

During diagnostic laparoscopy a number of accessory instruments are essential. These are instruments that must be placed through a second cannula unit. Surgical laparoscopy often requires a vast array of instruments designed for specific indications. Certain specialized instruments include stapling devices are generally 10mm or larger in diameter. Many of the biopsy and surgical instruments also have capabilities for monopolar electrosurgery at their distal tip.

AEM Laparoscopic Instruments: Shielded and monitored to prevent stray electrosurgical burns. Unintended tissue damage resulting from stray electrosurgical burns during laparoscopy can cause patient injury and may result in serious postoperative complications, even death. AEM laparoscopic instruments, based on excision's patented AEM technology, eliminate stray electrosurgical burns due to insulation failure and capacitive coupling.

What are stray electrosurgical burns?

During laparoscopy, stray electrosurgical burns can occur to non-targeted tissue, outside the surgeon's field-of-view (see Zones 2 and 3 in the figure below).

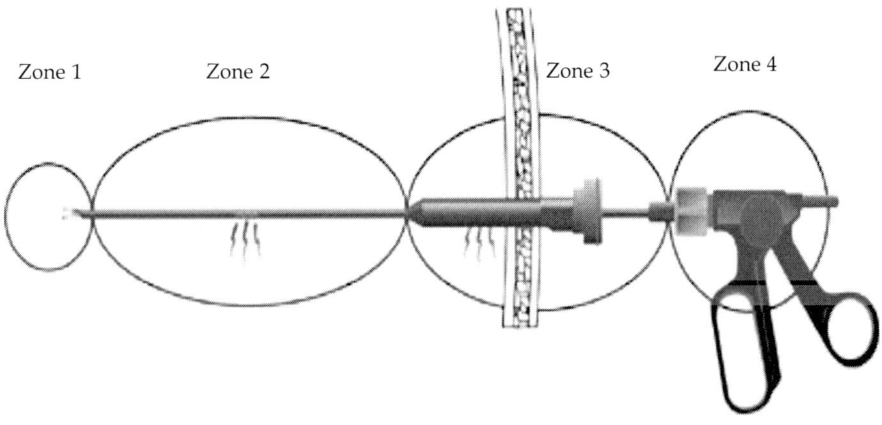

Once these burns have occurred they are often difficult to catch and diagnose. It may be several days before the patient returns to the physician complaining of severe abdominal pain. Postoperative complications due to stray electrosurgical burns include peritonitis and sepsis, conditions that can result in death.

Instrumentation for laparoscopy

(A) Instrument used for visualization of the abdominal cavity

- Light source (halogen/xenon).
- Fibreoptic light cable.
- Digital video camera.
- Digital video captures systems with floppy or compact disc.
- Medical grade colour monitor.
- Laparoscope (size 2.7 mm or 5 mm for small animals and 10 mm for large animals).

(B) Instruments for performing laparoscopy

- Veress needle for creating pneumo/capnoperitoneum.
- CO_2 insufflators automatically regulated for pressure and flow rate.
- Gas insufflation tubing.
- Trocar and cannula [primary (10-12mm), secondary and tertiary (5-8mm)].
- Laparoscopic scissors.
- Atraumatic grasping forceps.
- Smooth forceps designed for grasping the tubes.
- Bipolar and unipolar electrocoagulator.
- High flow irrigation-aspiration system.
- Needle holders
- Endoclip forceps.
- Endoclips and staples

(C) Instruments for laparoscope guided biopsy

- Instrument used for basic laparoscopy is the same for the biopsy except it requires additional different type of biopsy forceps, e.g. grasping, cutting etc.

(1) *5 mm Scissors and biopsy forceps*

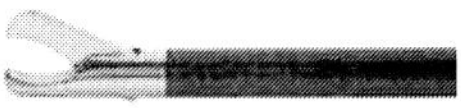

Hook scissors - single action, insulated shaft and handle, RF (Rotatable, fixed)-connector, (substitute - non-insulated shaft and handle)

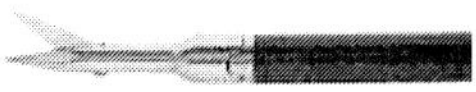

Micro tip scissors, straight, double action, non-insulated shaft and handle (substitute - insulated shaft and handle, RF-connector)

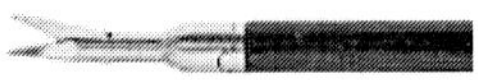

Micro tip scissors, curved, double action, non-insulated shaft and handle (substitute - insulated shaft and handle, RF-connector)

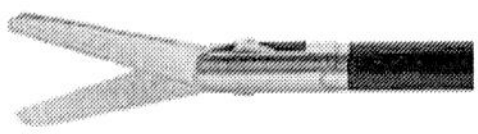

Metzenbaum scissors, straight, long blade, insulated shaft and handle, RF-connector

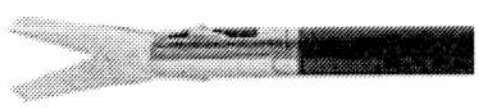

Metzenbaum scissors, straight, short blade, insulated shaft and handle, RF-connector

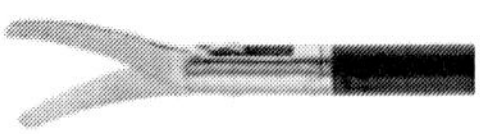

Metzenbaum scissors, curved, long blade, insulated shaft and handle, RF-connector

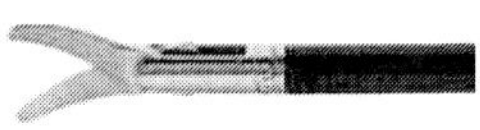

Metzenbaum scissors, curved, short blade, insulated shaft and handle, RF-connector

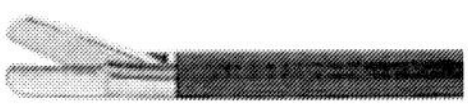

Peritoneal scissors - single action, non-insulated shaft and handle

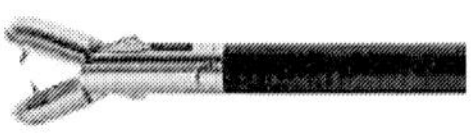

Biopsy spoon forceps, with tooth (Semm type), double action, insulated shaft and handle, RF-connector

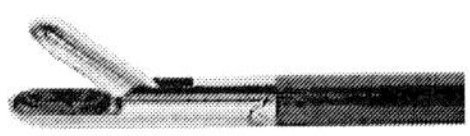

Biopsy spoon forceps - single action, non-insulated shaft and handle with spring.

(2) *Graspers*

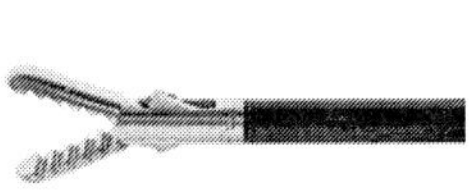

Aggressive backbiting grasper, insulated shaft, non-insulated ratchet handle, (substitute-insulated ratchet handle with RF-connector)

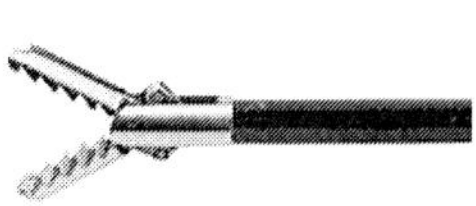

Alligator grasper - retro facing teeth, double action, insulated shaft, non-insulated ratchet handle, (substitute - insulated ratchet handle with RF-connector)

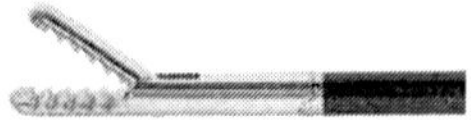

Alligator grasper - retro facing teeth, single action, insulated shaft, non-insulated ratchet handle, (substitute - insulated ratchet handle with RF-connector)

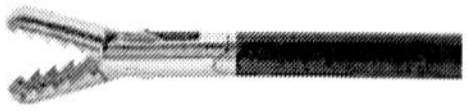

Cup shaped grasper/dissector - with teeth, double action, insulated shaft and handle, RF-connector

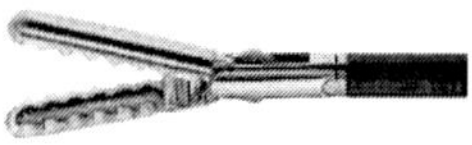

Wave grasper - long beveled edge jaw, double action, insulated shaft, non-insulated ratchet handle, (substitute - insulated ratchet handle with RF-connector)

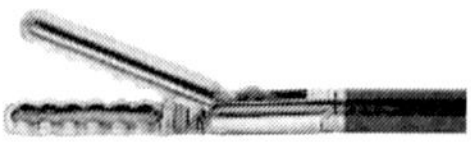

Wave grasper - long beveled edge jaw, single action, insulated shaft, non-insulated ratchet handle, (substitute - insulated ratchet handle with RF-connector)

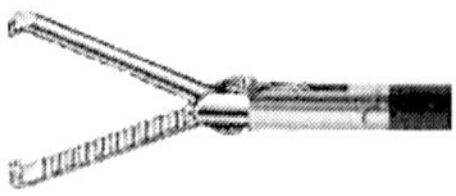

Retraction grasper, long ridged jaws, 2 x 3 atraumatic teeth, double action, insulated shaft, non-insulated ratchet handle, (substitute - insulated ratchet handle with RF-connector)

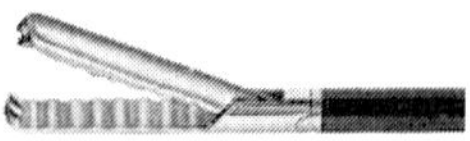

Retraction grasper, long ridged jaws, 2 x 3 atraumatic teeth, single action, insulated shaft, non-insulated ratchet handle, (substitute - insulated ratchet handle with RF-connector)

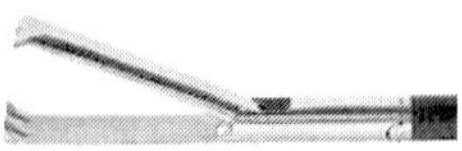

Claw grasper, 2 x 3 teeth, single action, insulated shaft, non-insulated ratchet handle, (substitute - insulated ratchet handle with RF-connector)

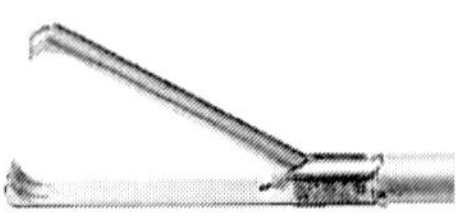

Claw grasper, 2 x 3 teeth, single action, non-insulated shaft, non-insulated handle with spring (substitute - insulated shaft)

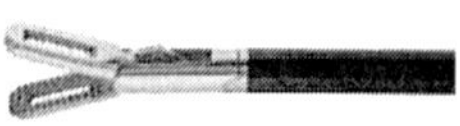

Fenestrated grasper, 16 mm double action jaw, insulated shaft, non-insulated ratchet handle, (substitute - insulated ratchet handle with RF-connector)

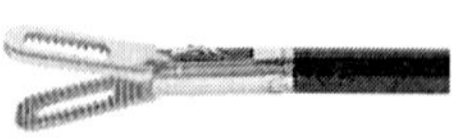

Fenestrated grasper, 22 mm double action jaw, insulated shaft, non-insulated ratchet handle, (substitute - insulated ratchet handle with RF-connector)

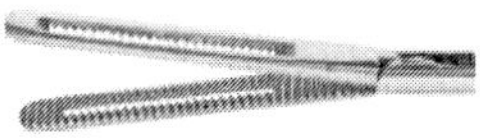

Fenestrated grasper, 40 mm double action jaw, insulated shaft, non-insulated ratchet handle, (substitute - insulated ratchet handle with RF-connector)

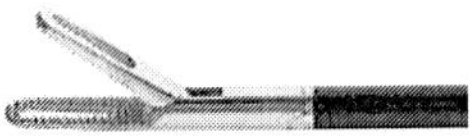

Johan fenestrated grasper, 22 mm single action flat jaws, insulated shaft, non-insulated ratchet handle, (substitute - insulated ratchet handle with RF-connector)

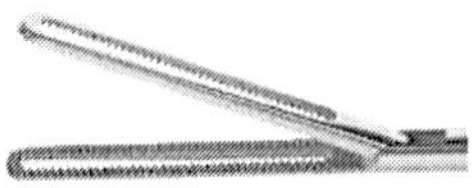

Johan fenestrated grasper, 40 mm single action flat jaws, insulated shaft, non-insulated ratchet handle, (substitute - insulated ratchet handle with RF-connector)

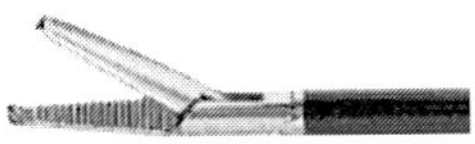

Kocher grasper, 1 x 2 teeth, single action, insulated shaft, non-insulated ratchet handle, (substitute - insulated ratchet handle with RF-connector)

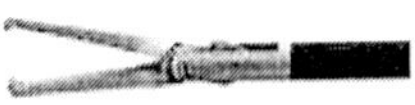

Kocher grasper, 1 x 2 teeth, double action (Weck type), insulated shaft, non-insulated ratchet handle, (substitute - insulated ratchet handle with RF-connector)

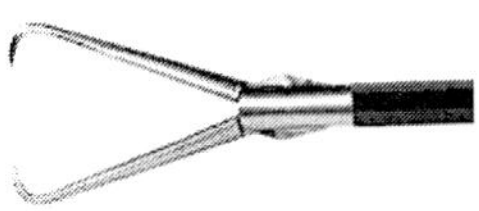

Schroeder tenaculum grasper, single tooth, insulated shaft, non-insulated ratchet handle, (substitute - non-insulated shaft)

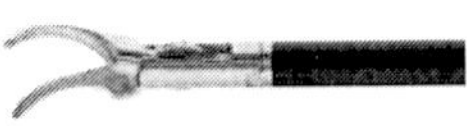

Kelly grasper/dissector, insulated shaft and handle, RF-connector

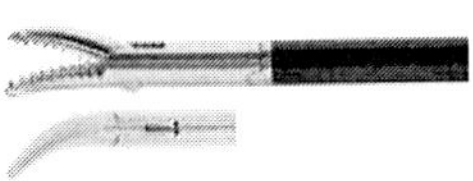

Petelin dissector, angled 60° left, single action, uninsulated shaft and handle, with spring

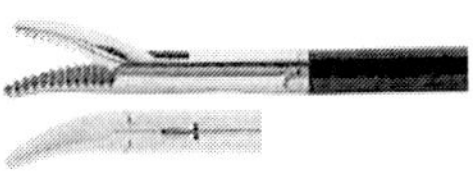

Petelin dissector, angled 30° left, single action, uninsulated shaft and handle, with spring

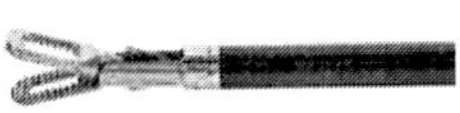

Micro grasper/dissector - fenestrated, insulated shaft and handle, RF-connector

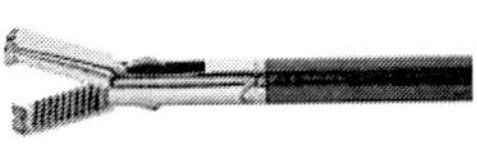

Cobra grasper - double action, insulated shaft and handle,RF-connector

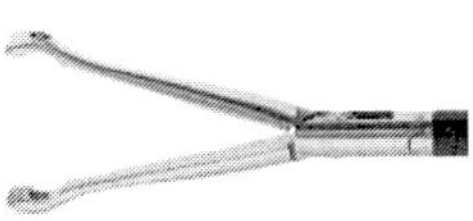

Babcock grasper - fenestrated tip, insulated shaft, non-insulated ratchet handle, (substitute - insulated ratchet handle with RF-connector)

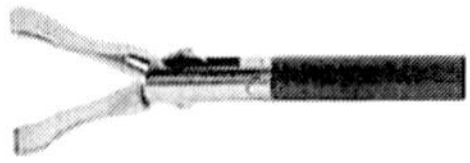

Babcock grasper - short version, delicate application, insulated shaft, non-insulated ratchet handle, (substitute - insulated ratchet handle with RF-connector)

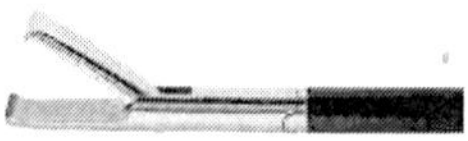

Allis grasper - short version, single action, insulated shaft, non-insulated ratchet handle, (substitute - insulated ratchet handle with RF-connector)

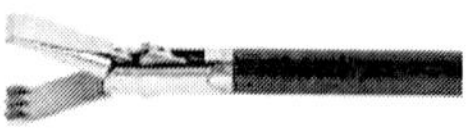

Allis grasper - short version, double action, insulated shaft, non-insulated ratchet handle, (substitute - insulated ratchet handle with RF-connector)

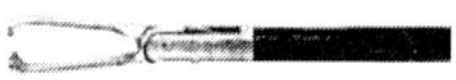

Allis grasper - medium version (Weck style), insulated shaft, non-insulated ratchet handle, (substitute - insulated ratchet handle with RF-connector)

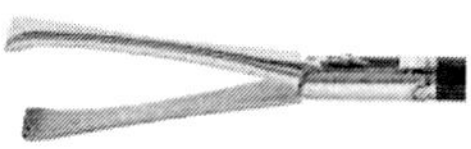

Allis grasper - standard version, insulated shaft, non-insulated ratchet handle, (substitute - insulated ratchet handle with RF-connector)

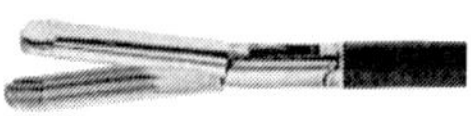

DeBakey grasper, 20 mm Jaw length, insulated shaft, noninsulated ratchet handle, (substitute-insulated ratchet handle with RF-connector)

(3) *5mm Grasping and dissecting forceps*

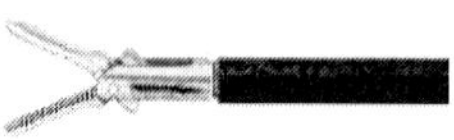

Micro Reddick-Olsen grasper/dissector, insulated shaft and handle, RF-connector

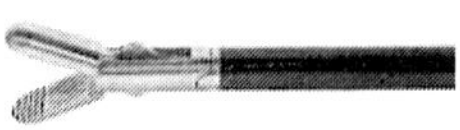

Standard grasper, with spoon, insulated shaft and handle, RF-connector

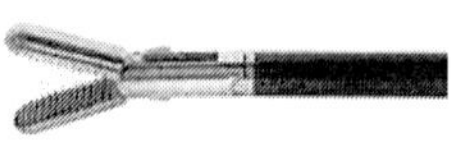

Standard grasper, insulated shaft and handle, RF-connector (Substitute - insulated or non-insulated ratchet handle)

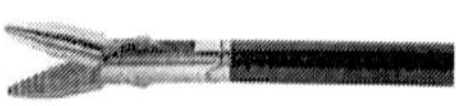

Bullet-nose grasper/dissector, with spoon, insulated shaft and handle, RF-connector

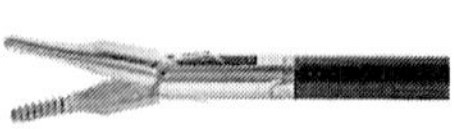

Tapered dolphin-nose grasper/dissector, insulated shaft and handle, RF-connector

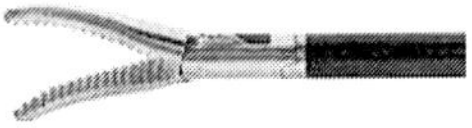

Maryland grasper/dissector, insulated shaft and handle, RF-connector

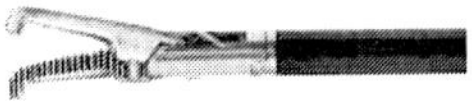

Mixter grasper/dissector - right angle, insulated shaft and handle, RF-connector

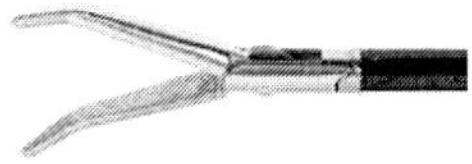

Mixter grasper/dissector, 45° Angle, insulated shaft and handle, RF-connector.

Cleaning and sterilization of laparoscopic instruments

Laparoscopic surgery required expensive surgical instruments that are inherently difficult to clean. Steam sterilization in an autoclave is not possible for many instruments and ethylene oxide sterilization is either unavailable or unsuitable between operations in many instances. The commonest method seems to be the use of prolonged exposure to formaldehyde gas in a chamber or immersion in glutaraldehyde.

It is recommended that certain laparoscopic instruments such as optics that cannot be sterilized in an autoclave should receive a high level of disinfections. Decontamination of instruments should be done immediately after surgery by thorough washing and the use of an ultrasonic cleaner. The latter are now easily available in India. Instruments that can be taken apart must be disassembled prior to washing.

Formaldehyde has a broad spectrum of action on micro-organisms. A number of studies have shown that with contact time of 60-180 minutes, formaldehyde at 0.2% will only sanitize. Formaldehyde at 2% will disinfect and will sterilize. Formaldehyde works best at a relative humidity of >80% and at higher temperatures and its activity against spores and acid-fast bacilli is slow. The use of glutaraldehyde is effective, but the manufacturer's instructions regarding pH, self-life, and time for disinfections or sterilization must be followed.

In general, manufactures will instruct veterinarians on appropriate cleaning and care of laparoscopic instruments. On completion of each procedure, laparoscope and accessories should be cleaned according to the manufacture's instruction. Following laparoscopy the telescope, cannula, trocar, Veres needle and all other accessory instruments should be washed in luke warm water and dried prior to storage. Some of the accessory instruments of the laparoscopic unit are not autoclavable. Gas sterilization is an effective and safe procedure for the laparoscope and accessory instruments. Most common method of sterilization is immersion in a disinfectant solution. Ten to fifteen minutes of immersion in activated dialdehyde is sufficient to prevent infection. Immersion in chlorhexidine is also effective. Rinsing the instruments with sterile water prior to use is essential.

Decontamination, cleaning, high-level disinfectant and chemical sterilization of laparoscopes

Laparoscopes are delicate instruments that must be handled with great care to prevent damage. The following recommendations will help to protect these instruments and prolong their use. Laparoscopes and accessories should be sterilized or high-level disinfected using chemical agents. Glutaraldehyde and formaldehyde are the best chemical high-level disinfectants for soaking laparoscopic instruments because they do not damage rubber, plastics or lens cements. Other high-level disinfectants, such as 6% hydrogen peroxide, may be corrosive.

How to decontaminate and clean laparoscopes after use

STEP 1 : Immediately after use, gently wipe the laparoscope, fiber-optic light source and cable and plastic tubing with luer-lock with a cloth soaked in 60–90% ethyl or isopropyl alcohol to remove all blood and organic material.

STEP 2 : Completely disassemble the laparoscopic equipment: operating laparoscope, trocar, scissors, forceps, Veres needle, needle holder and clip applicator etc.

STEP 3 : Place disassembled parts in a basin of clean water and mild, nonabrasive soap.

STEP 4 : Wash all outer surfaces, using a soft cotton cloth.

STEP 5 : Clean inner channels with a cleaning brush supplied with the laparoscope kit. Use a circular motion to remove particulate matter (organic matter hidden in the narrow channels may cause infection later). Be careful not to forcibly push the brush against the closed end of the inner tube as this may damage it.

STEP 6 : Rinse all parts thoroughly with clean water three times. Use the brush to remove soap and particles from the inner channels. (Soap, if not thoroughly rinsed away, will decrease the effectiveness of the disinfectant).

STEP 7 : Dry equipment with a clean soft cotton cloth or air dry. (Excess water will dilute the disinfectant and decreasing its effectiveness).

STEP 8 : Clean lenses at least weekly, and more often as needed, but do not touch the lenses with fingers.

STEP 9 : High-level disinfect (for 20 minutes) or sterilize (overnight), or if not needed immediately, carefully store in instrument container after cleaning and drying until next use.

Instrumentation and procedures

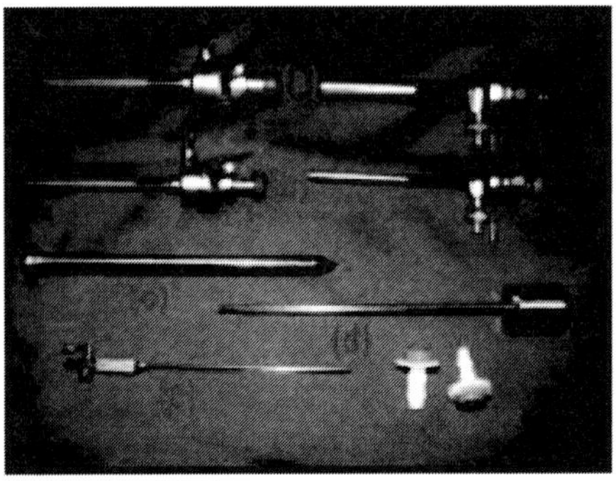

Instruments for laparoscopy (a) 10 mm cannula (b) 5 mm cannula (c) 10 mm pyramidal tip trocar, (d) 5 mm safety trocar, (e) Veress needle (f) Adapter

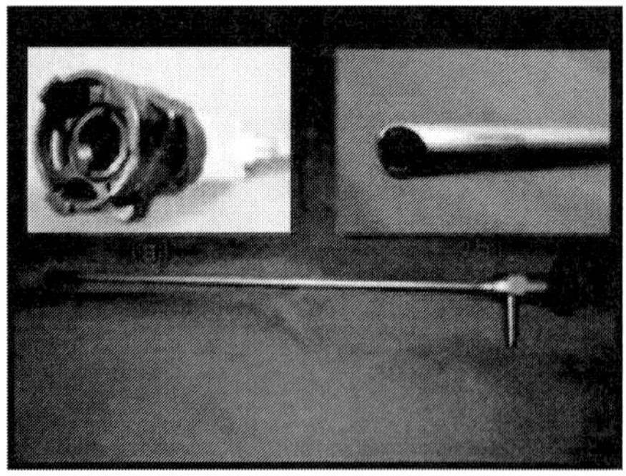

5 mm 30 forward-oblique telescope (a) Endocamera (b) Telescope tip

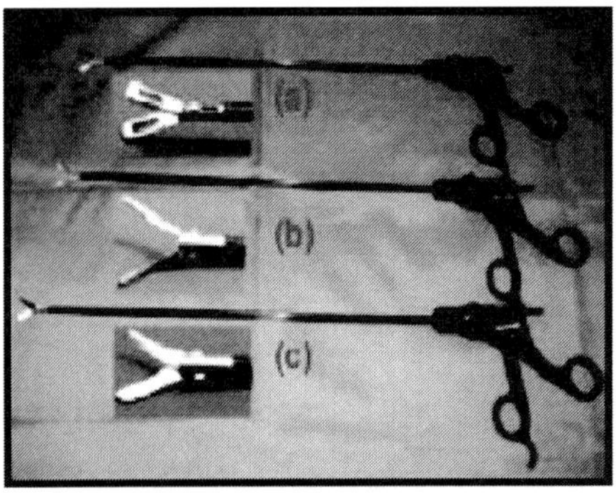

Laparoscopic instruments (a) Fenestered grasping forceps, (b) Traumatic forceps, (c) Monopolar scissors

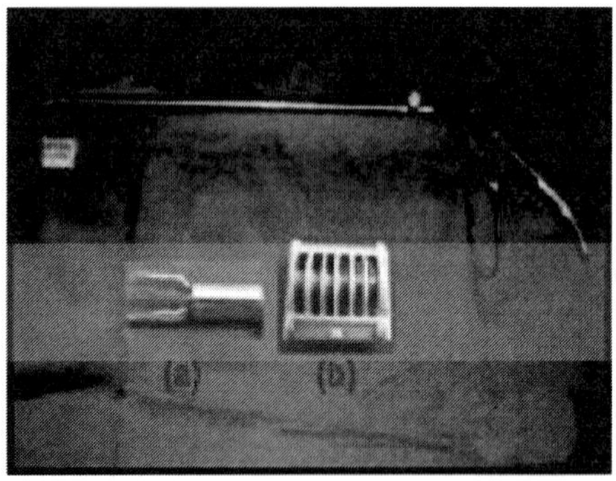

Endoclip applicator (a) Tip of clip applicator (b) Titanium clip cartridge

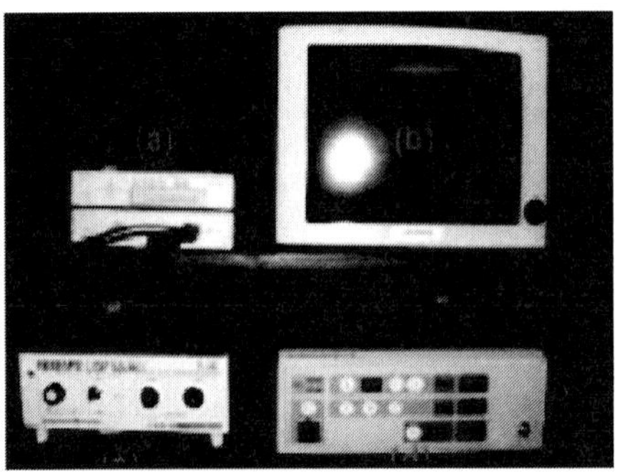

Laparoscopic equipment's
(a) L-cap, (b) Television monitor (c) Halogen light source, (d) Endoflator

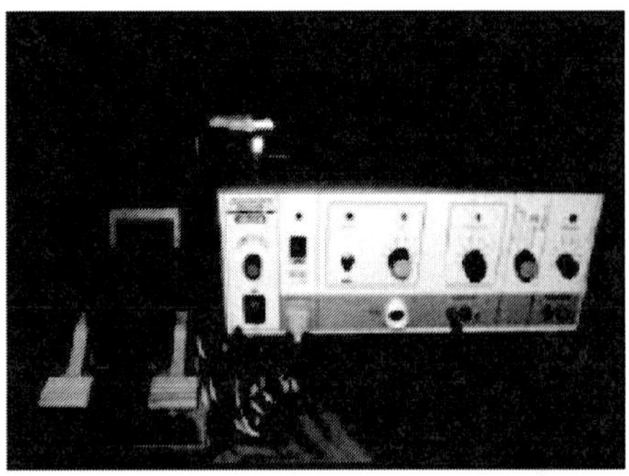

Electrocautery unit

Instrumentation and procedures

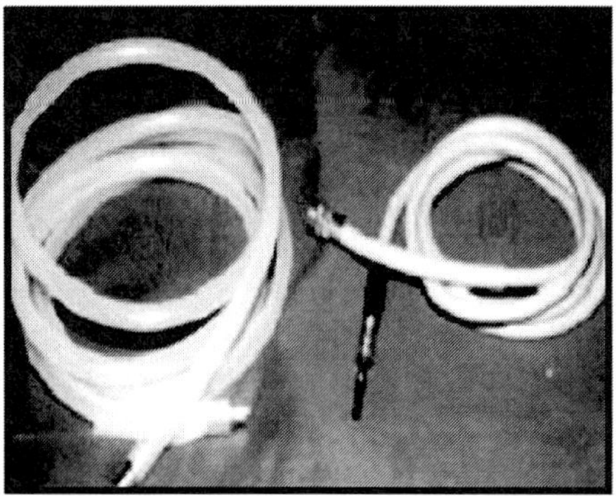

Laparoscopy equipment's (a) CO_2 gas hose, (b) Fibre optic cable

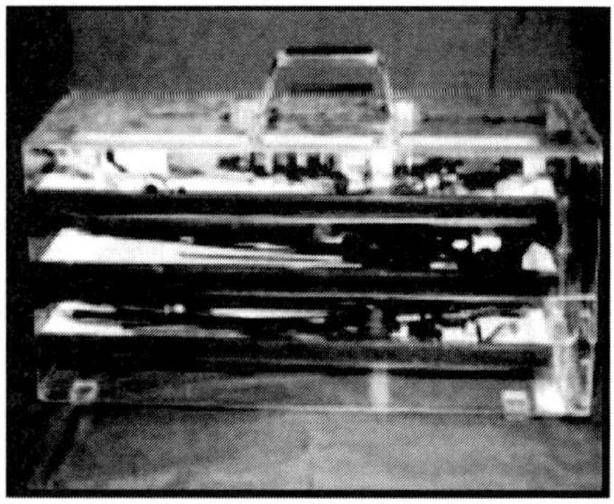

Closed formalin chamber

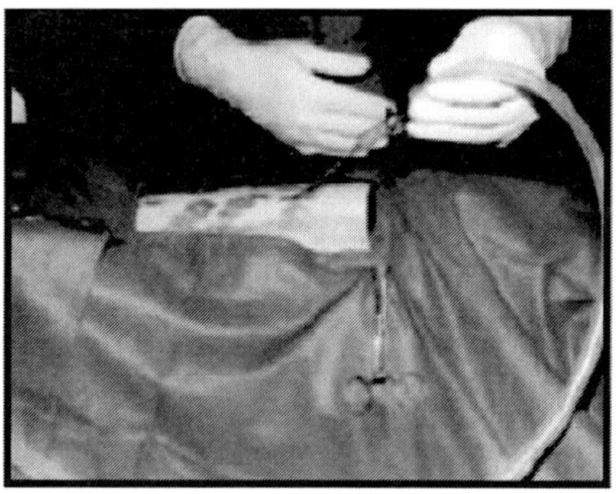

Insertion of Veress needle

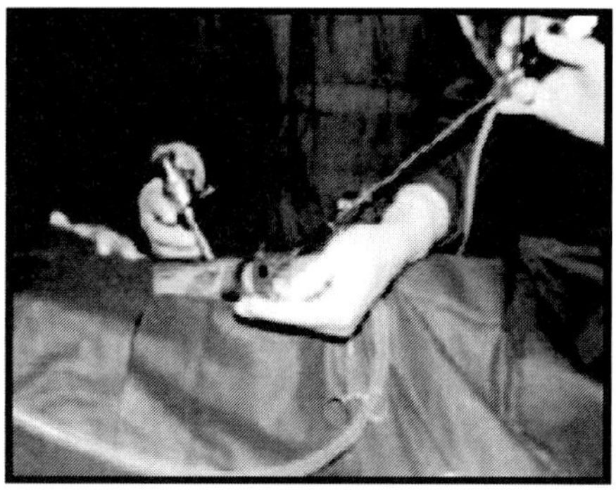

Outside arrangement of three trocars

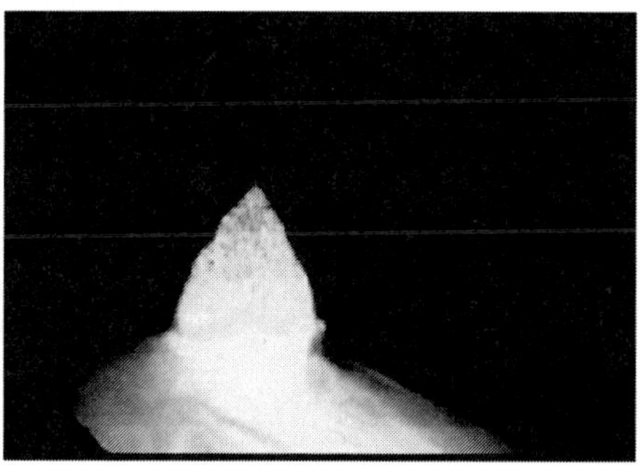

Entry of trocars under laparoscopic guidance

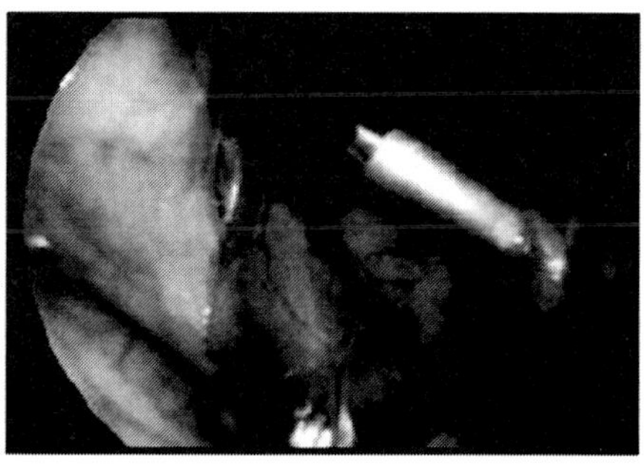

Entry of trocars under laparoscopic guidance

How to clean lenses on laparoscopes

STEP 1 : Remove the plastic eyepiece of the laparoscope prior to cleaning the proximal lens with acetone or 60–90% alcohol. (Acetone and other organic solvents can severely damage plastic).

STEP 2 : Clean lenses with a cotton swab soaked in alcohol or acetone. (Cotton will not scratch the lens and alcohol and acetone will not weaken the cement around the lens).

STEP 3 : While cleaning, do not touch lenses with fingers. (Skin oils may damage the lenses).

STEP 4 : Clean lenses at least weekly, and more often as needed.

How to sterilize laparoscopes

STEP 1 : Decontaminate, wash and dry all instruments to be sterilized as described above.

STEP 2 : In a well-ventilated area, wearing gloves to prevent skin irritation, completely immerse clean, dry, disassembled instruments and cleaning brush in a plastic container at least 8 cm (3 inches) in depth that contains either 8% formaldehyde or 2–4% glutaraldehyde (e.g., Cidex®). The disinfectant must touch all surfaces in order to be effective.

Note: Avoid placing instruments on top of each other, as this may damage them.

STEP 3 : Cover the container during the disinfection procedure. (This will decrease the rate of evaporation and will keep dust out of the solution).

STEP 4 : Allow soaking 8 to 10 hours in glutaraldehydes, and at least 24 hours in formaldehyde. Both agents work best at room temperature. Sterilization cannot be assured at temperatures less than 20^{0}C (68^{0}F). Because instructions vary, carefully read manufacturer's instructions for each product.

STEP 5 : Use sterile gloves to carefully remove the instruments from the solution (Forceps or lifters may damage the instruments).

STEP 6 : Rinse three times with sterile water to completely remove all traces of the disinfectant. If sterile water is unavailable, rinse in cold water which, has been filtered and boiled for 20 minutes. Use a sterilized or high-level disinfected brush to assist with rinsing the narrow channels of the instruments. (This keeps movable parts from sticking due to any remaining disinfectant.) Finally, rinse completely with 60–90% ethyl or isopropyl alcohol. Allow to dry and use immediately. Do not store laparoscopes that have been rinsed with alcohol because residue can cause movable parts to stick.

STEP 7 : Air dry in a sterile container with a cover. (Laparoscopes and accessories can be stored for up to 1 week in this container).

How to high-level disinfect laparoscopes

STEP 1 : Decontaminate, wash and dry all items to be high-level disinfected.

STEP 2 : In a well-ventilated area and wearing gloves to prevent skin irritation, completely immerse clean and dry disassembled instruments in a plastic container containing either 8% formaldehyde or a 2– 4% glutaraldehyde (e.g. Cidex) solution. The disinfectant must touch all surfaces in order to be effective.

Note: Avoid placing instruments on top of each other, as this may damage them.

STEP 3 : Cover the container during the HLD process. (This will decrease the rate of evaporation and will keep dust out of the solution).

STEP 4 : Allow soaking for 20 minutes.

STEP 5 : After 20 minutes, use high-level disinfected or sterile gloves to carefully remove instruments from the solution. (Forceps or lifters may damage the instruments).

STEP 6 : Rinse three times with cold water that has been filtered and boiled for 20 minutes in order to completely remove all traces of the disinfectant. (This will prevent the solution from irritating the client's skin and keep the movable parts from sticking). Although not necessary, sterile water can be used in place of boiled water. Use a high-level disinfected brush to assist with rinsing the narrow channels of the instruments.

STEP 7 : Allow to air dry in a high-level disinfected container or dry with a high-level disinfected soft cotton cloth and place immediately on the instrument table.

How to store laparoscopes

STEP 1 : Decontaminate, wash and dry all instruments to be stored.

STEP 2 : Assemble laparoscope and trocar.

STEP 3 : Place laparoscope and trocar in the padded container supplied with the equipment and store in a cool, dry place. *Remember*: Before using stored laparoscopes and accessories such as trocars, they must be disassembled, cleaned and either sterilized or high-level disinfected.

Tips for prolonging the life of laparoscopes

- Failure to completely disassemble and clean the laparoscope properly is the most common cause of problems. In addition, blood and other organic material left to dry on the instruments is difficult to remove and may be a source of infection.
- Never autoclave or boil laparoscopes because heat will damage the optics. Always sterilize or high-level disinfect with chemical sterility or disinfectants such as glutaraldehyde or formaldehyde.
- Remove instruments from the disinfectant solution as soon as timing requirements are met. Prolonged immersion may shorten the life of the instrument.
- Rinse at least three times with sterile cold (or boiled) water after cold sterilization or high-level disinfection respectively, to remove residue. Residue can cause movable parts to stick.
- Wear sterile or high-level disinfected gloves to handle instruments after final processing.

- Avoid picking up or handling instruments in groups or bunches.
- Always grasp the telescope at the eyepiece end to avoid damaging the operative forceps.
- Avoid piling instruments on top of each other to prevent damage or fiber breakage.
- Do not use Savlon as it is not a high-level disinfectant and has been associated with clouding laparoscope optical lenses.

❑❑❑

4

Anesthesia

Anaesthesia is an important criterion for doing laparoscopic procedure, which is being achieved by induction of general anaesthesia. However, in certain species, e.g. bovine, caprine etc., it can be done by preanaesthetic agent and infiltration of the local anesthetic agent at the site of the trocar placement. Selection of an anesthetic agent depends on the patient conditions, nature of procedure; time to be taken for the laparoscopic procedure and available facility. For the induction of the general anaesthesia follow the same procedure as in the conventional surgery viz. fasting, water withheld, preanaesthetic, fluid administration etc. Further, due to difference in the physiology of cardiopulmonary system of different animals, all these considerations varied from species to species and breed-to-breed. For instance cattle and buffalo are more prone to regurgitation and subsequent aspiratory pneumonia in general anaesthesia than those of dog and cat. While going for induction of general anaesthesia, an anesthetist should know about the different drug being used, their mechanism of action, effect on the different body system, their adverse effect and pure antagonist, if possible. Besides this an anesthetist should also know about the patient physiology and equipment for the administration of the anesthetic agents, because veterinary anesthetist is faced with numerous disturbances of cardiopulmonary and skeletal muscle function associated with general anaesthesia. For anaesthesia no anaesthetic agent is safe until and unless it is used by an experienced anesthetist.

Once the decision is made to perform laparoscopy there are a number of pre-surgical details and considerations to be made. The patient should be fasted for at least 12 hours before the procedure and the urinary bladder should be evacuated. If the stomach or urinary bladder is distended there is an increased risk of traumatic puncture with either the trocar or Veress needle and they will hinder the view of the internal organs.

In abroad, laparoscopy is commonly performed using general gas anaesthesia. Most patients tolerate general anaesthesia well during laparoscopy however, it is expected that the pneumoperitoneum from CO_2 insufflation will increased intra-abdominal pressure and may interfere with excursions of the diaphragm. Recent studies have found that in most cases that although the PaO_2 concentrations decrease and $PaCO_2$ concentrations increase these physiologic changes are generally considered to be minimal and within physiologically accepted limits. It is advised to avoid high intra-abdominal insufflation pressures or excessive tilting of the surgical table that would apply undue pressure from the abdominal organs on the diaphragm. In cases in which ventilation becomes compromised it will become necessary for assisted ventilation.

A brief account of the general anaesthesia in different animals is given below:

Cattle and buffalo

Cattle are not good subject for heavy sedation or general anaesthesia, especially in lateral or dorsal recumbency because of following problem/complications:

- Regurgitation followed by the aspiration of ruminal contents in the lungs.
- Bloat caused by failure in the eructation process due to ruminal content filled in the esophageal orifice.
- Due to pressure over diaphragm by abdominal viscera, ventilation becomes shallow, rapid and inefficient for gas exchange within the lungs.

These complications can be minimized by :

- With holding all food for 24 h to 48 h and water for 8 to 12 h before anaesthesia.
- When the animal in lateral recumbency during anaesthesia the head should be lower than the general body level so that saliva and any regurgitated material runs freely from the mouth.

- Leave the endotracheal tube in the trachea with the cuff inflated until the animal is in sternal recumbency.

Tracheal intubations are not mandatory for all sedated or anaesthetized recumbent bovine animals since regurgitation is not always occurring. Anticholinergic drugs e.g. atropine sulphate, glycopyrrolate and scopolamine are not of much use for they make the secretion more viscid in nature and not significantly reduce its production. For biopsy procedure performed in standing position, only sedation and local analgesia is sufficient.

The different drugs used for the tranquilizer/sedation are as follows:

- Triflupromazine hydrochloride (Siquil®, Sarabhai)- 20 mg/100kg body weight, i.m.
- Acepromazine hydrochloride -0.4 to 0.6 mg/kg, i.m.
- Diazepam hydrochloride (Calmpose®)- 0.05 to 1.0 mg/kg, i.m.
- Xylazine hydrochloride - 0.20 to 0.50 mg/kg, i.m.

General anesthesia in cattle and buffalo can be induced by premedication with xylazine (0.10-0.20 mg/ kg, i.m.) followed by ketamine hydrochloride @ 2 mg/kg, i.v. chloral hydrate 30-60 g and 10% halothane after tracheal intubations can also be used.

Sheep and Goat

As in the cattle, sheep and goat also have a problem of regurgitation and respiratory distress during the general anaesthesia. Tracheal intubation is difficult due to narrow jaw. Withhold the food for 24 h and water for 6-12 h before anaesthesia. Lamb and kid should be prevented from sucking for 30-60 minutes before anaesthesia. Following drug combination may be used for general anaesthesia in sheep and goat.

- Diazepam hydrochloride @ 0.20 to 0.30 mg/kg, i.v. and ketamine hydrochloride @5.0 to 7.5 mg/kg, i.v. (10 to15 minutes).
- Xylazine hydrochloride @ 0.10mg/kg and ketamine hydrochloride @ 6mg/kg, i.v. or 11 mg/kg, i.m. (30 minutes). Additional

dose of xylazine hydrochloride can be given if the depth of anaesthesia is not adequate.

- Thiopental sodium @ 7 to 20 mg/kg, i.v. for a short period of anaesthesia (10 minutes).
- Xylazine hydrochloride @ (0.10 mg/ kg, i.m.) and tiletamine-zolazepam @ 4 mg/kg, i.v. (45 to 60 minutes).

Equine

In horses sedation and anaesthesia can be produced by the administration of the xylazine @ 1.1 mg / kg, i.v. and xylazine @ 1.1 mg/kg, i.v. + ketamine hydrochloride @ 2.2 mg/kg, i.v. respectively.

Swine

In pig 6-8 h fasting and 2 h water withholding is necessary. Atropine sulphate- 0.30-2.4 mg/kg i.v. or i.m. (total dose) '!Xylazine @1mg/kg i.m. and Azaperone @ 1-2 mg/kg i.m. wait for 20 minutes, then endotracheal intubation '! then Thiopental sod (2.5%) 5-10 mg/kg i.m. or i.v. Muscle relaxant suxamethonium 2.8 mg /kg or alcuranium 0.10 mg /kg may be required during the anaesthesia because pig muscle have much tonicity than other animals.

Dog and cat

Ketamine is probably the best anaesthetic agent in the pre-anaesthetized dogs and cats due to its less cardiopulmonary complication. Ketamine produces best anaesthesia with atropine sulphate (0.045mg/kg, s.c. or i.m.), diazepam (0.5mg/kg, i.v.) and/ or xylazine (0.5mg/kg, i.v.) combination. For optimum effect, ketamine and diazepam are administered separately at an interval of 10 minutes. Simultaneous intravenous administration after mixing the solution in one syringe has also been recommended. This combination provides surgical anaesthesia for a minimum period of 15-20 minutes. Xylazine produces emesis in dog therefore; Ketamine should be injected after emesis, if occurred. Ketamine (0.1% solution in 5% dextrose) in premedicated patient (atropine and acepromazine) can be used as intravenous drip for induction (120-150 drop/minute) and maintenance (15-30 drop/minute) of general anaesthesia. In cat

0.2 mg/kg midazolam and 10mg/kg ketamine mixed in same syringe and administered i.m. produced heavy sedation with good muscle relaxation. Induction by thiopental sodium (2.5- 5.0%) can be used in dogs and cats premedicated with the either diazepam (0.50 mg/kg i.v.) or midazolam (0.2-0.30 mg /kg i.v.) and maintenance by 3.5% halothane after endotracheal intubations. In common practice, animals are fasted for 24 hours before anaesthesia. Animals are premedicated with atropine sulphate at 0.04 mg/kg subcutaneously. After 10 minutes, general anaesthesia is achieved with a combination of xylazine hydrochloride at 1mg/kg and ketamine hydrochloride at 10mg/kg intramuscularly.

Zoo/Laboratory animals and wildlife

For zoo/laboratory animals xylazine and ketamine is the best sedative and to induce the general anaesthesia halothane or isoflurane can be used after tracheal intubations. For wildlife, restraining may be achieved by either etorphine or carfentanil. These agents are very dangerous and to meet out any emergency or overdosing anatagonist like diprenorphine or atipamezole should be available with such drugs.

Avian laparoscopic procedures require administration of general anaesthesia. Many different anesthetic regimens have been used for birds. Isoflurane gas anaesthesia has become the standard for avian anaesthesia since its introduction to the field in the mid 1980's. A number of parenteral agents, either singly or in combination, have been used such as ketamine, xylazine, diazepam midazolam and propofol. Perhaps, none of these agents has proven to be as safe or consistently effective as isoflurane for endoscopic/laparoscopic procedure. Ketamine @ 20 mg/kg body weight, i.m. provide suitable restraint for laparoscopic examination. Ketamine (0.5 mg/kg)-xylazine (0.01mg/kg) combination provides smooth induction and recovery. Placing a soft, uncuffed endotracheal tube into the glottis readily intubated birds. Remember that in most avian species the tracheal rings are complete. For rat and rabbit, xylazine and ketamine are used at a rate of 5mg/kg and 50mg/kg intramuscularly respectively.

❑❑❑

5
Laparoscopic Procedures

Positioning of the patient/ anesthesia

The patient is transported to the operating room and after general anesthesia the patient is placed in a desirable position. Some operating tables can be repositioned intraoperatively, allowing the surgeon to change the angle of the patient during the procedure. Special care should be taken to avoid nerve injury by malpositioning the patient, particularly along the popliteal fossa and brachial plexus. If any part of the patient is in contact with a metal object, patient may be at risk of electro surgical burns. General anesthesia is preferred for laparoscopy as it provides adequate muscle relaxation and assisted respiration particularly as the patient is in Trendelenburg position.

Position of the operating team and equipments

The laparoscopic surgeon must be familiar with the mechanics and operation of each piece of equipment. Prior to anesthetizing the patient the operating team must check that the insufflator is functioning and has an adequate supply of gas. The light source is functioning and the video equipment is in working order. This will prevent avoidable malfunctions, which may result in serious complications and surgical delays. Mobile racks for camera and TV monitor, video-recorder, light-source and insufflators should available which, helps in organization of the operating room equipment.

The surgeon stands on the left side of the patient and the assistant on the opposite side. From here, the surgeon is able to continuously monitor all of the equipments (insufflators, light-source, irrigation system, electric generator). Alternatively, the surgeon and his assistant may both stand to the left of the patient with the video monitor on the opposite side. The TV monitor (1 or 2) should be located so that each member of the operating team may follow the procedure. If there is only one monitor, it is best placed at the feet of the patient.

Pneumoperitoneum

The first step in laparoscopy is to establish a pneumoperitoneum before cannula placement. The begins with placement of the Veress needle either adjacent to the cannula portal sites or in the same site to be used by the first telescope portal.

Insert the "Veress" needle through a vertical, 1cm intraumbilical incision. In general a 7cm length is sufficient although a 15cm needle is also available for very obese patients. Prior to insertion the spring mechanism of the needle is checked to avoid visceral puncture. At intraumbilical site the abdominal wall is thinnest with no intervening fat and the peritoneum closely underlying the fascia.

To insert the 'Veress' needle the abdominal wall is lifted with one hand and the needle passed through the incision. Once the needle as it passes through the abdominal wall, one should always assure that the Veress needle is actually in the abdominal cavity and is not retained in the muscle planes of the abdominal wall or has penetrated an organ. Inadvertent insufflation in the subcutaneous tissues with CO_2 makes the procedure almost impossible to continue. To assure that the Veress needle is in the abdominal cavity and not within an organ the "hanging drop test" can be performed. This requires placing a drop of saline in the hub of the Veress needle and then lifting the abdominal wall with the needle shaft, the negative pressure within the abdominal cavity will pull the drop of saline into the needle. This then assures that the needle is in the correct location. Insufflation of gas into a mass, organ or vessel can result in fatal air emboli. The Veress needle is then attached to the automatic CO_2 insufflator. When the abdomen is adequately distended with CO_2, it will become tympanic upon palpation.

Insufflate carbon dioxide at a flow rate of 2 L/minute, allowing the patient to adapt gradually to the pneumoperitoneum. When a pressure of 12 mmHg is obtained, place the machine on automatic flow in order to maintain this pressure. Most machines will automatically adjust the flow rate (usually at a maximum flow of 6 L/min.). The abdominal pressure should be no greater than 15mmHg and in most all cases 10-12 mmHg is adequate to maintain abdominal distention and perform laparoscopy in small animals.

Authors studied the effect of different carbon dioxide pressure gradients in capnoperitoneum/pneumoperitoneum for laparoscopic examination in dogs. The physiological effects are pronounced over 14mmHg of CO_2 pressure gradient. Marked increase of respiration rate in correlation with increased pCO_2 and decreased pO_2 are observed. Myocardial ischemia or hypoxia as reflected through S-T segment depression is observed at 14mmHg pressure gradient. Physiological stress is remained significantly higher with 14 mmHg intra-abdominal pressure.

Placement of trocar

After attaining a sufficient pneumoperitoneum, place one 10-12 mm trocar with cannula through the Veres needle incision. During insertion of the trocar, compress the upper abdominal wall with the free hand to make the lower abdominal wall tense, giving a firm platform against which to insert the trocar and cannula. Direct the trocar towards the pelvis to avoid injury to major vessels. The trocar should pierce the peritoneal cavity as high as possible to assure a panoramic view. Occasionally, the trocar may be placed above the umbilicus (this should be done under direct laparoscopic visualization through an initial umbilical site).

After confirming the correct positioning of trocar and cannula unit withdraw trocar and insert the laparoscope through the cannula and immediately confirm correct intraperitoneal placement. Standard diagnostic laparoscopes vary in diameter from 5-10mm. The 5mm laparoscope is adequate for inspection but is not sufficient for more complex procedures. The light source is also an essential element. In general the standard 150 watt light source is sufficient only for diagnostic laparoscopy. Complex procedures require a more powerful light (250-400 watt halogen lamp).

Positioning and site of laparoscopy in the different animals

Animal	Anaes-thesia	Position	Site	Procedure
Dog and Cat	Xylazine-Ketamine	Supine/ Dorsal	For laparoscope- Ventral midline caudal to umbilicus. For Trocar-Lateral to right and left rectus abdominis muscle	Intestine and jejunum biopsy.
		Dorsal recum-bency (Trendele nburg)	-do- (4 trocar in abdominal wall)	Ovariohysterectomy
		- do -	Midline hole 2-4 cm cranial to the umbilicus, for trocar- 6-8 cm lateral to the first hole.	For the direct observation of the internal organs (ovary, uterine horn, urinary bladder, spleen, liver (right medial lobe right lateral lobe and caudate lobe), and gall bladder. Jejunum, descending colon and ventral portion of colon, ventral portion of each kidney.
Buffalo / Cow	Sedation + local anaes-thesia	Standing	Right Para lumbar fosa (upper and lower third)	Observation of ovary
Sheep and Goat	General Anaes-thesia	Trendelen burg	Right side below the umbilicus and rib cage- 5 cm anterior to umbilicus and 5 cm to the right of the midline	For the liver, kidney biopsy
Calf	Sedation + local anaes-thesia	Standing	Right PLF (Center of PLF and 4 cm caudodorsal from the first site)	Liver biopsy
Horse	Sedation + local anaes-thesia	Standing	-	Ovariectectomy
	General Anaes-thesia	Recum-bency	-	Castration

Next, place the patient in Trendelenburg position in order to allow the gravitational effect to move the bowel out of the pelvic cavity. Then insert two or three 6 mm trocar and cannula units under direct vision at ancillary puncture sites for instruments. These secondary units are inserted supra pubically, taking care to avoid the epigastric vessels laterally and the bladder medially.

Collaboration with the anesthetist

The pressure of the pneumoperitoneum and the extent of the Trendelenburg position must be adapted to the haemodynamic and respiratory demands of each individual patient. Continued communication and collaboration with the anesthetist throughout the procedure is mandatory. This is extremely important because it may be necessary to reduce the Trendelenburg position, lower the intra-abdominal pressure, or even convert to laparotomy at any time during the procedure.

Closure of abdominal incisions

After completing the laparoscopic procedure remove the ancillary ports and examine the incisions internally for bleeding. Then remove the laparoscope and allow the intra-abdominal gas to escape through the sleeve. Take the patient out of Trendelenburg position in order to optimize the decompression of the pneumoperitoneum. Close the incisions with non-absorbable sutures. It is wise to place an absorbable fascial suture in the larger >10 mm umbilical incisions followed by a cutaneous non-absorbable suture.

❑❑❑

6

Techniques for Laparoscopic Examination

Laparoscopy is an operative procedure designed for the visual inspection of peritoneal cavity and biopsy of organs. Laparoscopy is a valuable diagnostic and therapeutic tool in clinical medicine. In the field of cholecystectomy, appendicectomy, vagotomy, hernia repair and adhesion release laparoscopy surgery offers significant advantages over open surgery in humans. For gynecological problems like ovarian cyst or in the case of oophorectomies and hysterectomies, laparoscopic surgery ('scarless surgery') is now considered a better alternative in addition to laparoscopic sterilization. Only in the last 15 years laparoscopy is widely used in different animal species for research and clinical diagnostic and therapeutic purposes. The first canine laparoscopy procedures were performed in the early 1900's (Kelling, 1902). Anderson (1937) used dogs to perfect his skills prior to human clinical trials. The first clinical application of laparoscopy in dog's involved ovarian function studies in the early 1960's and Lettow reported the first laparoscopic liver biopsy procedure in a dog in 1972.

Indications

- Direct visual examination of the various abdominal structures including peritoneum, diaphragm, liver, gall bladder, kidney, spleen, pancreas, ovaries, urinary bladder, stomach and intestines.
- Diagnosis of early or ectopic pregnancy.
- Liver biopsy.

- Cholecystocentesis.
- Kidney biopsy.
- Intestinal biopsy.
- Adrenal evaluation.
- Splenic evaluation.
- Reproductive evaluation.
- Feeding tube placement.
- Gastropexy.
- Surgical breakdown of adhesions.
- Cholecystocholangiography.
- Gastric foreign body removal.
- Cryptorchid surgery.
- Cystoscopy.
- Tube cystotomy.
- Splenic pulp pressure measurement.
- Laparoscopic ovariohysterectomy-bilateral oopherectomies, uterine horn ligation or occlusion or ovarian coagulation in the female.
- Laparoscopic vasectomy-vas deferens occlusion in males.
- Detection of ovarian or paraovarian cyst.
- Pregnancy diagnosis.
- Embryo collection.
- Laparoscopic sexing in monomorphic birds.

Instrumentation

The basic equipment for performing laparoscopy includes the laparoscope/telescope and corresponding trocar and cannula, light source, gas insufflator and the Veress needle. Laparoscope applicable for use in the small animals (dog, goat, sheep and lab animals) ranges from 1.7 to 10 mm in diameter, however, a 5mm diameter telescope is suitable for most cases and 2.7mm may be required for toy breeds of dogs and lab animals. A 0 or 30 degree direction of vision provides the operator with a "normal' field of view and has proven most useful. The trocar-cannula size corresponding to the diameter of the laparoscope should be used. Trocar tips are either conical or pyramidal. The pyramidal tip is preferred because it facilitates easier abdominal wall penetration. The cannula consists of a hollow channel to accommodate the telescope with a valve, which prevents insufflation loss while removing the trocar or inserting the laparoscope/ telescope. A light source containing a 150 Watt lamp is sufficient for routine diagnostic laparoscopy. A flexible fibre optic cable is required to transmit light source to the laparoscope. A flexible 6 mm fibreoptic light transmitting cable is generally advocated for dog to provide more light transmission and hence, better internal illumination. The Veress needle is a spring-loaded, blunt-tipped needle used to establish a pneumo/capnoperitoneum. A Veress needle of 120mm length and equipped with an on-off luer-lock adapter is suitable for use. Automatic gas (CO_2) insufflator provides a great deal of convenience and safety during laparoscopic examination by allowing measurement of total gas volume delivered as well as intra-abdominal pressure. Other equipments and instruments used are standard ones.

Animal preparation

Animals should be fasted for at least 12 hours before laparoscopy and water should be withheld in the morning of the procedure. The urinary bladder, stomach and colon ideally should be empty. If the stomach or urinary bladder is distended there is an increased risk of traumatic puncture with either the trocar or Veress needle and they will hinder the view of the internal organs.

Anaesthesia and restraint

Laparoscopy in the small animals is performed in surgical plane of anaesthesia. It can be done under local anaesthesia in certain situations, but in conjunction with tranquilizers or narcotic analgesics. In severely depressed patients, local anaesthesia may be sufficient. Barbiturates anaesthesia should be avoided in cases of hepatic insufficiency, as well as ketamine in dogs with renal insufficiency. Inhalation anaesthesia may be instituted if necessary. Intramuscular injection of ketamine hydrochloride (10.0 mg/kg) and xylazine (1 mg/kg) to produce anesthesia is the choice of anaesthesia for laparoscopic diagnosis and laparoscopy guided-biopsy in dogs. The combination of ketamine (5-10 mg/kg i.v.) and diazepam (0.1 mg/kg i.v.) may also be used. Atropine is routinely used as a pre-anaesthetic. In goats, xylazine @ 0.1mg/kg i.m. and ketamine @ 5-6mg/kg i.v. or 10 mg/kg i.m. for 30 minutes are used. Additional dose of xylazine can be given if the depth of anaesthesia is not adequate. In laboratory animals, thiopental (2.5%) @ 5-10 mg/kg i.v. or xylazine @ 0.5 mg/kg. i.m. and ketamine@ 5mg/kg. i.m. is the choice of anaesthesia for laparoscopic diagnosis and laparoscopy guided-biopsy. In some situations the authors are performed diagnostic laparoscopy using only heavy sedation in conjunction with local anaesthesia at the entry sites. In quick short diagnostic procedures or in the severely depressed patients this is often work adequately or in conjunction with short acting intravenous anaesthesia.

Procedure

The selection of a midline, right or left lateral abdominal approach depends on the organs to be examined or manipulated. The right lateral approach is used routinely for diffuse hepatopathies, right-sided liver masses, pancreatic biopsy, right kidney and adrenal biopsy. This approach allows visualization of the caudate, right lateral, right medial, and quadrate lobes of the liver as well as the gall bladder, common bile duct, descending duodenum, right limb of the pancreas, pylorus, diaphragm, right kidney and small intestine. A left lateral abdominal approach is utilized in animals with left-sided liver masses, for splenic visualization and biopsy, splenoportography, measurement of splenic pulp pressure, visualization of left kidney and adrenal gland. A ventral mid-line approach has also been preferred by some veterinarians, however, falciform fat in the anterior ventral abdomen sometimes obscure visualization.

The objective of the laparoscopy procedure must be determined in order to select the appropriate cannula portal placement sites. The two most common approaches include the right lateral and a midline approach. The right lateral approach is the recommended approach for diagnostic evaluation of the liver, gallbladder, right limb of the pancreas, duodenum, right kidney and right adrenal gland. A ventral approach is often useful for many operative procedures, and offers good visualization of the liver, gallbladder, pancreas, stomach, intestines, reproductive systems, urinary bladder and spleen. In the ventral approach the primary portal is placed on or adjacent to the midline near the umbilicus. A disadvantage of the ventral approach is the falciform ligament that may hinder visualization of the anterior abdomen especially in obese animals. A left lateral approach may be used, but because the spleen lies directly under the normal entry sites the potential for splenic trauma by a trocar is a likely possibility. With any approach, the entry site may be modified by moving either cranial or caudal to assure adequate working space for the laparoscope and for the procedure to be performed.

The animal is placed on the operating table in either left or right lateral recumbency. A table that can be tilted to shift abdominal viscera is recommended, since this can enhance visualization of peritoneal organs. The animal's limbs are secured to the table to prevent movement during the procedure. Any movement may damage the precious laparoscopic instruments. Surgical sterility is maintained throughout the procedure. The area is clipped, surgically scrubbed, disinfected and draped.

The first step in laparoscopy is to establish a pneumoperitoneum before cannula placement. This begins with placement of the Veress needle either adjacent to the cannula portal sites or in the same site to be used by the first telescope portal. Generally the needle is inserted in the lower abdominal quadrant, 4-6 cm lateral to the midline. The underlying structures should be palpated before insertion the needle. After insertion, the needle is swept gently in a circular pattern to free any adhesions or omentum that might interfere with insufflation. Once the needle as it passes through the abdominal wall once should always assure that the Veress needle is actually in the abdominal cavity and is not retained in the muscle planes of the abdominal wall or has penetrated an organ. Inadvertent insufflation in the subcutaneous tissue with CO_2 makes the procedure almost impossible to continue. To assure that the Veress needle is in the abdominal cavity and not within an organ the "hanging drop test" can be performed. This requires placing a drop of saline in the hub of the Veress needle and then lifting the abdominal wall with the needle shaft the negative pressure within the abdominal cavity will pull the drop of saline into the needle. This then assures that the needle is in the correct location. Insufflation of gas into a mass, organ or vessel can result in fatal air emboli. The veress needle is then attached to the automatic CO_2 insufflator. The CO_2 gas hose from the endoflator/insufflator is attached to the luer-lock of the Veres needle and a moderate pneumoperitoneum/capnoperitoneum is established using a flow rate of approximately 1 liter/minute to a final abdominal pressure of approximately 10-12 mm Hg. The required insufflation volume depends on the animal's body size. Respiration and capillary perfusion should be closely monitored, since over distention can lead to cardiopulmonary compromise. When the abdomen is adequately distended with CO_2 it will become tympanic upon palpation. The abdominal pressure should be no greater than 15 mm Hg.

Midline technique

After achieving sufficient pneumoperitoneum/capnoperitoneum a 1-2 cm midline incision is made in the skin 2-4 cm cranial to the umbilicus. The trocar- cannula unit is held at 30^0 to the longitudinal plane of animal and inserted through the incision into the abdominal cavity. The trocar-cannula unit is passed through the abdominal wall using a twisting and thrusting motion. One will hear a hollow "pop" and the sound of hissing air through the trocar once it has entered the gas distended abdomen and immediately after abdominal entry the sharp trocar is removed from the cannula to prevent possible organ trauma. The trocar is removed and the gas hose pipe` from Veress needle is attached to the cannula. Following the initial cannula placement the telescope is prepared for entry into the abdomen. The light cable is then attached to the telescope and the light guide cable attached to the light source. A video camera is next attached to the telescope and focused to give a sharp clear image. The telescope is now advanced through the cannula and into the abdomen. Frequently the image will becomes blurred as it enters the abdominal cavity is either due to tissue fluid or blood contaminating the lens due temperature change, particularly during cold weather. When this occurs, remove the telescope from the abdomen and kept the tip of the telescope in hand palm for few minutes and then simply cleaned with povidone iodine or using saline soaked gauze and re-entered into the abdominal cavity. Once the telescope is in the abdominal cavity, careful examination of the contents is performed. Next the site of entry for the second/accessory portal is selected. This location depends on the ancillary procedures that are to be performed. The technique for placement of the accessory cannula involves visual laparoscopic control viewing the trocar entry from inside the abdomen. Once the approximate entry site is determined the abdominal wall is depressed with a finger and the site is viewed internally identifying the palpation site. The entry site is then assessed to assure that underlying organs will not be traumatized during trocar entry. The second cannula is then placed through the abdominal wall as described in the procedure for the first telescope cannula except one watch the trocar entry is viewed internally. Once the cannula has entered the abdomen the trocar is removed.

Lateral abdominal approach

After obtaining pneumoperitoneum a 1-2 cm (depending on the trocar size) skin incision is made on the ventrolateral abdominal wall at a variable distance caudal to the ribs. A typical entry site is 3-4 cm caudal to the last rib halfway between the ventral midline and lumbar vertebral transverse process. However, the exact position of the puncture site depends on the organ of interest and the size and body condition of the animal. The right lateral approach is used for diffuse or multifocal hepatopathies, right-sided liver mass and pancreatic biopsy, and biopsy of the right kidney or adrenal gland. This approach allows visualization of the caudate, right lateral, right medial and quadrate lobes of the liver as well as the gall bladder, common bile duct, descending duodenum, right limb of the pancreas, pylorus, diaphragm, right kidney and small intestine. A left lateral abdominal approach is utilized in left-sided liver masses, for splenic visualization and biopsy, splenoportography, measurement of splenic pulp pressure, visualization and biopsy of the left kidney or adrenal gland.

Examination of the viscera

The laparoscope should be warmed before insertion to prevent moisture condensation on the distal lens. This can be done by inserting the laparoscope tip in warm sterile saline or holding it in the palm for several minutes. Touching the tip gently against internal organs cleans "fogging" or contamination of the distal lens. Occasionally the laparoscope is withdrawn for cleaning with povidone-iodine. Commercial anti-fogging solutions are also available. The operator should begin viewing as soon as the laparoscope is placed within the cannula. Viscera immediately underlying the puncture site are inspected to identify the trauma or hemorrhage may be resulting from improper trocar insertion. The entire abdomen should then be systematically examined to detect any abnormalities.

Exploration of the abdominal cavity is assisted by using the palpation probe to "feel" and move the organs as needed. As the probe or any instrument is passed into the abdomen it should be viewed as it exits the cannula and it is then directed to the area of examination. Instruments should never be blindly passed into the abdomen but rather viewed internally as they pass through the cannula and directed to the area of interest. Using this technique will prevent serious tissue trauma by the probe or other accessory instruments.

Authors are routinely used this technique for direct examination of internal organs in different small animals. Laparoscopic examination is performed under surgical plane of anaesthesia. A drug combination of xylazine hydrochloride (0.1mg/kg) and ketamine hydrochloride (10mg/kg) is injected intramuscularly in goats. Dogs are anaesthetized by giving an intramuscular injection of xylazine (1mg/kg) and ketamine hydrochloride (5mg/kg), whereas rabbits are anaesthetized with same combination of drugs (xylazine 5mg/kg and ketamine hydrochloride 50mg/kg) given intramuscularly. All animals are fasted for 12-24 hr before laparoscopy and water is withheld on the morning of the procedure. The urinary bladder, stomach and colon are made empty before the procedure.

Laparoscopes and accessory instruments are kept in 2% glutaraldehyde solution for 30 min prior to use and rinsed in warm distilled water immediately before surgical use. Animals are placed on a surgical table and are restrained in a supine, head-down position at an angle of approximately 30 degree. The exploratory laparoscopy for visualizing and examining different abdominal organs is conducted at the ventral abdominal midline, 2-4 cm cranial to the umbilicus.

Capnoperitoneum/pneumoperitoneum is maintained at 10-12 mm of Hg pressure gradient.

Laparoscopy is used for direct observation of the reproductive tract to determine ovarian dynamics (ovulation, number of Graffian follicles, changes in the shape of the follicular dome and presence of corpus luteum). For observing reproductive tract, urinary bladder is to be first identified. In dogs, each vas deferens is easily located and fully observed from its origin to its descent through the abdominal inguinal ring. Uterine bifurcation and oviduct are also easily visible. The urinary bladder, liver, spleen, gall bladder, pancreas are observed in all animals. Tortuosity of urinary bladder is variable depending on the distension of the bladder. Spleen is visualized in the upper left abdominal quadrant, cranial to the left kidney. In the upper right abdominal quadrant, liver is identified by its bright red colour and uniform smooth surfaces. Gall bladder is visualized in between right medial and right lateral lobes and appeared as distended, round and bluish in colour, however, in rabbit it is elongated in shape. The stomach is appeared as dense, pale red in colour and is situated towards the mid-abdominal plane. Different parts of small and large intestine are also easily identified and the rectum appeared right to the urinary bladder with good visibility. Visualization of the pancreas, duodenal portion of small intestine is sometime difficult. It is also sometime difficult to distinguish the prostate in male dogs due to anatomical location, which vary with the position and volume of the urinary bladder. However, accessory probe is helpful to visualize these organs.

Laparoscopy technique is not only use for visualizing different normal abdominal organs in different animal species, but also it enormously useful to diagnose different intra-abdominal pathological lesions in animals.

Authors used this laparoscopic technique in many clinical cases of dogs after routine clinical and biochemical examination. Intra-abdominal pathologies including intestinal torsions, intestinal intussusceptions, intestinal adhesions, intestinal impactions, mummified fetus, polycystic ovarian and uterine growth, persistent corpus luteum, spleenomegaly, splenic abscess, splenic tumour, chronic hepatitis, cirrhosis, hepatomegaly, liposarcoma of liver and bridging fibrosis of liver are diagnosed by laparoscopic examination. Biopsy of the diseased organs is taken using laparoscopy and histopathology of laparoscopic biopsy samples is confirmed of different abdominal affections.

Termination of examination and postoperative care

At the conclusion of the laparoscopic procedure the instruments and telescope are removed and the pneumoperitoneum is allowed to escape. To obviate the possibility of postoperative pain, it is important to evacuate the gas as much possible. This is accomplished by the depressing the trumpet valve and allowing the CO_2 to escape from the cannula. Deflation can be facilitated by gentle massage of the ventral abdominal surface. The instruments are then removed, rinsed in trap water and returned to the germicidal soaking solution. Generally a single suture for the peritoneal layer and 2-3 sutures for the skin are used. The need to apply topical antibiotic ointment or to administer parenteral antibiotic depends on the measure of sterility maintained during laparoscopic examination. For postoperative pain management we generally infiltrate bupivacaine local anaesthesia in the trocar cannula sites and prescribe systemic analgesia.

Contraindications

- Cardio-pulmonary decompensation.
- Coagulopathies.
- Excessive intraabdominal adhesions.
- Profound ascites.
- Bacterial peritonitis.
- Diaphragmatic hernia.
- Inguinal hernia.
- Advanced cardiac diseases.
- Very small patient (less than 2kg body weight).
- Excessive intra-abdominal body fat.

Laparoscopic view of different peritoneal organs in goat

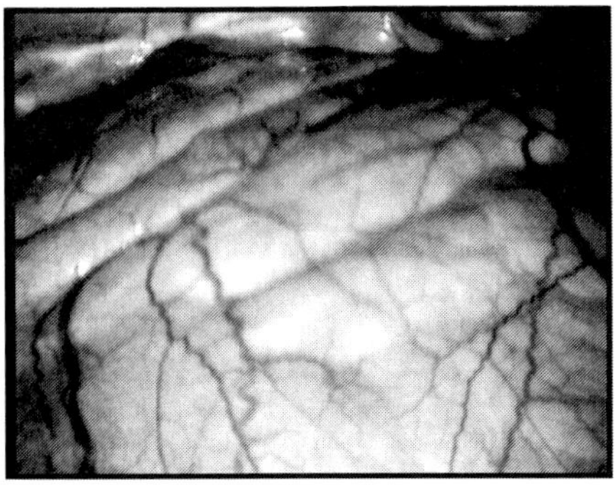

Small Intestine

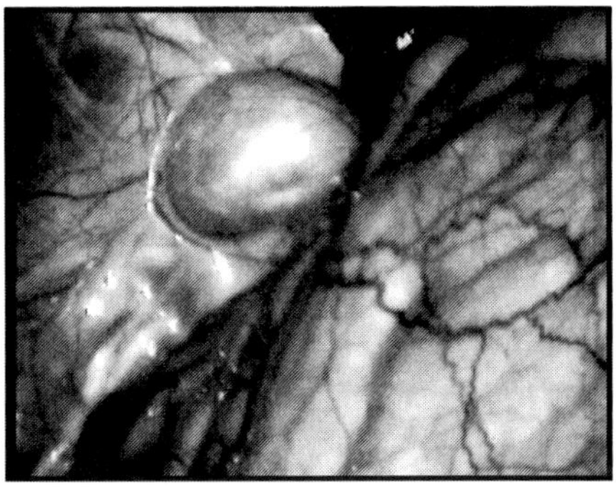

Kidney

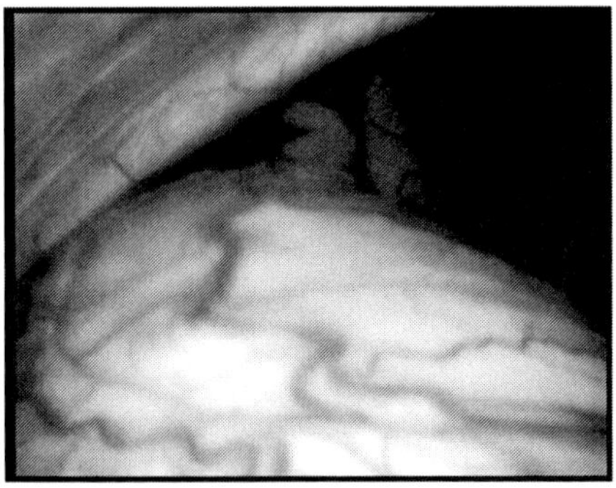

Urinary Bladder

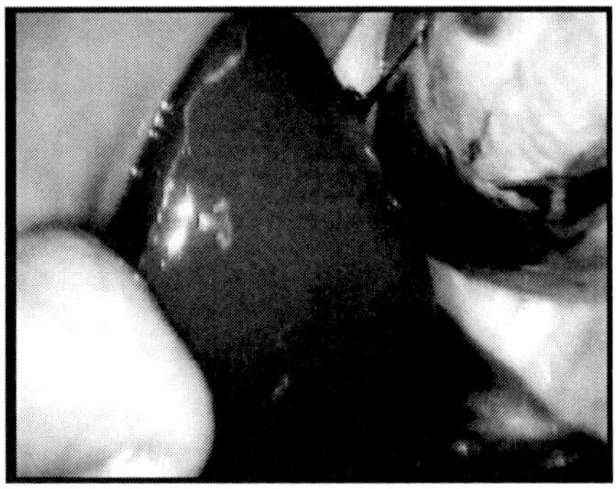

Liver

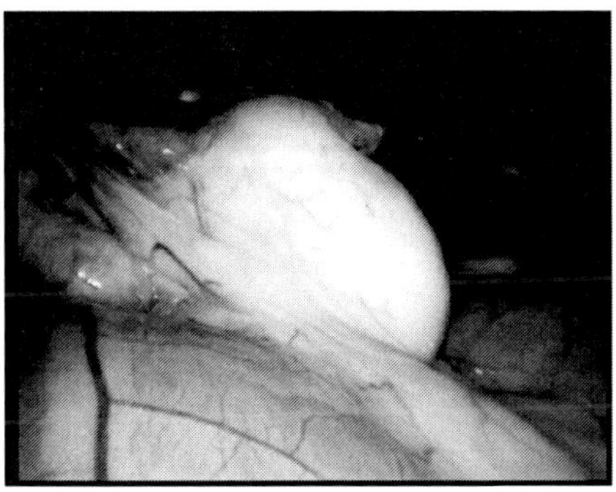

Gall Bladder

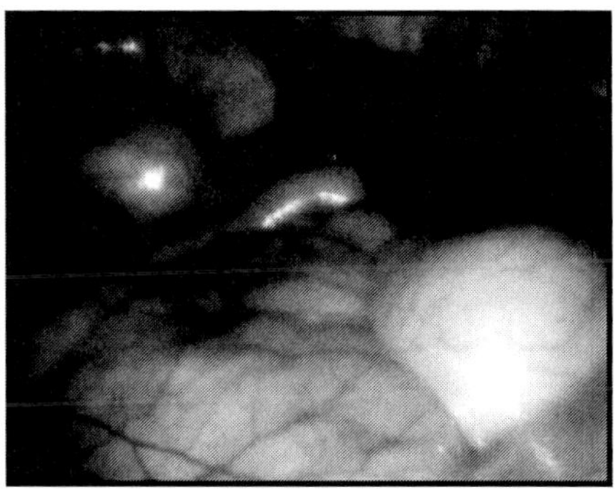

Abomasum

Laparoscopic view of different peritoneal organs in rabbit

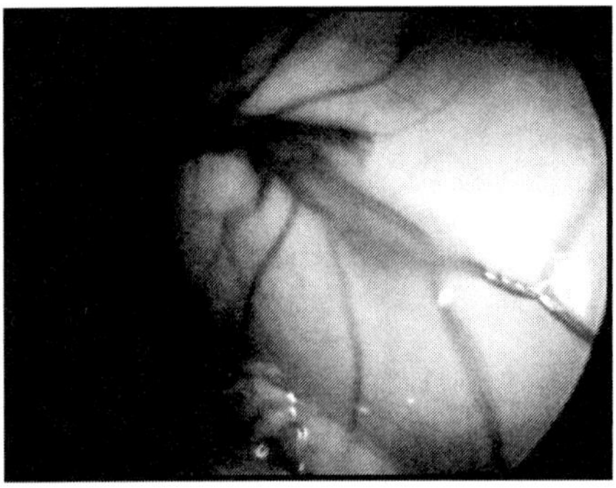

Stomach

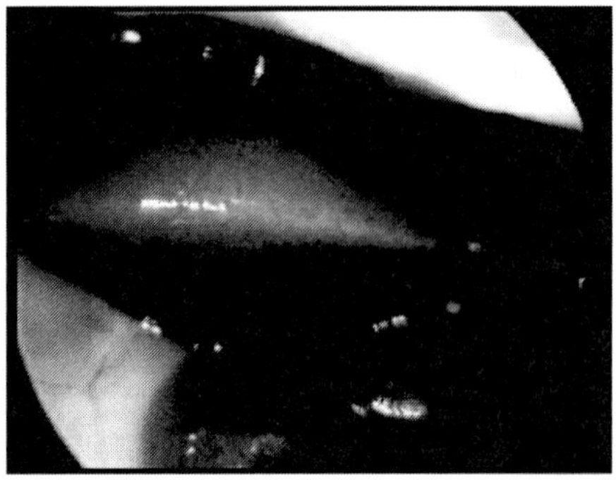

Liver

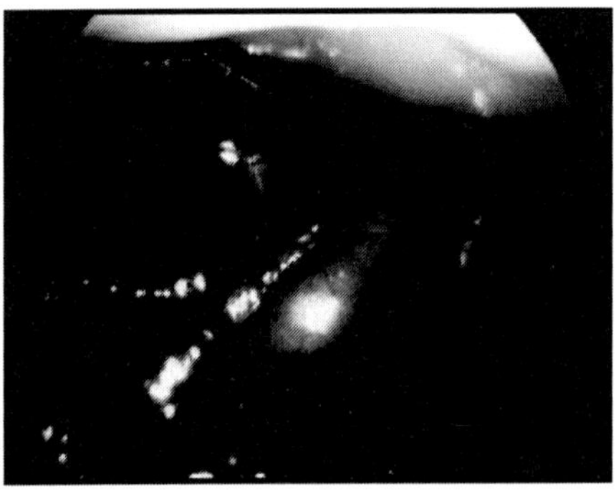

Gall Bladder

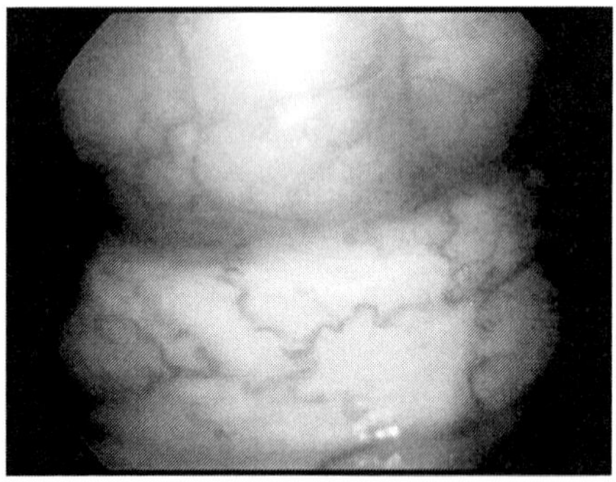

Urinary Bladder

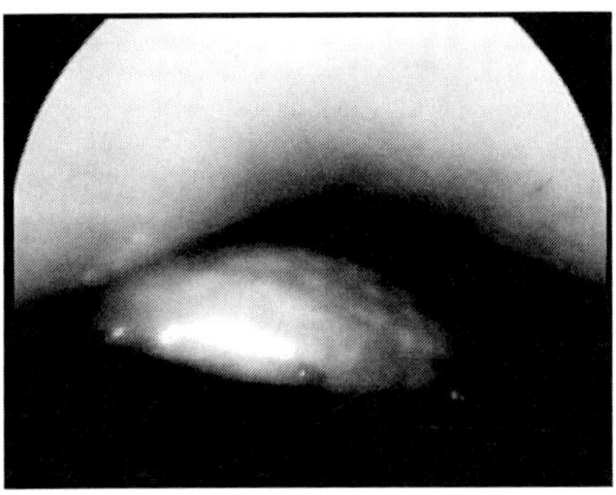

Spleen

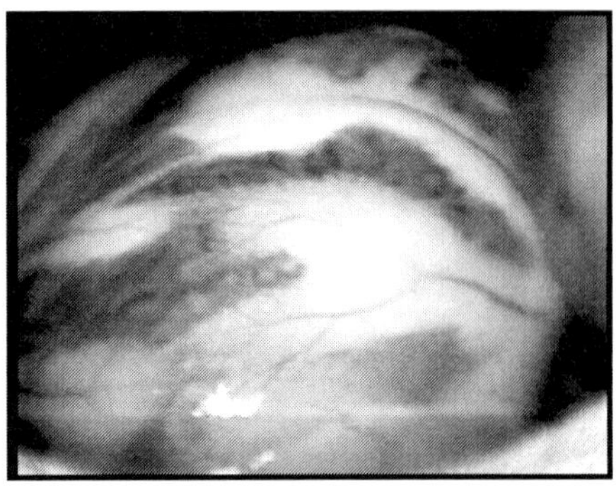

Large Intestine

Laparoscopic visualization of different organs in dog

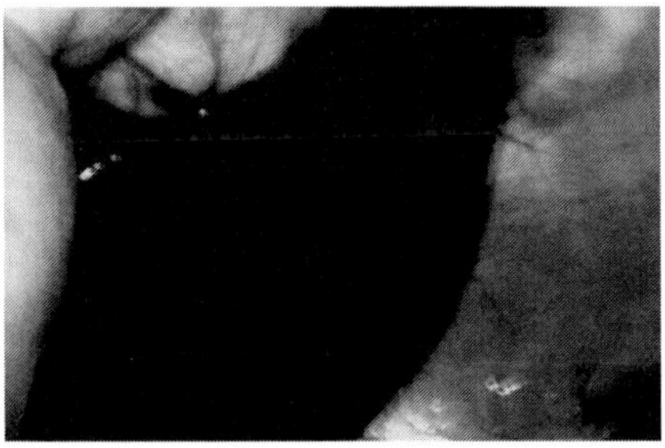
Liver

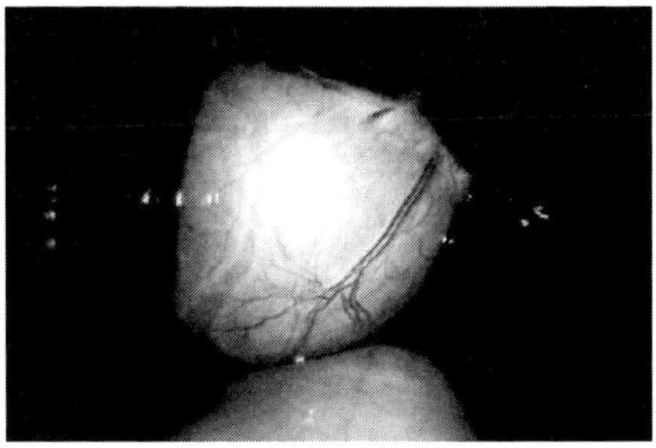
Gall Bladder

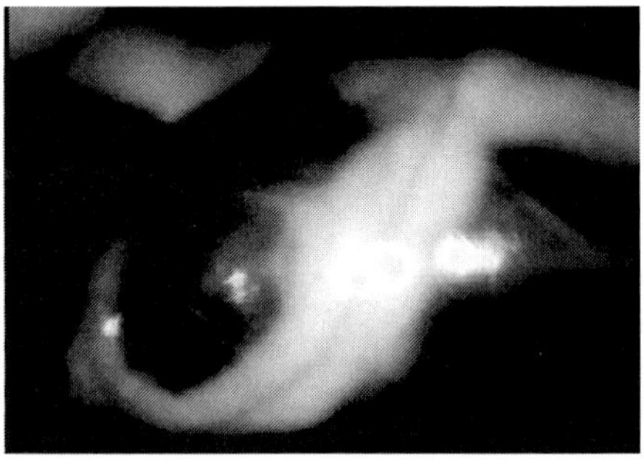
Kidney

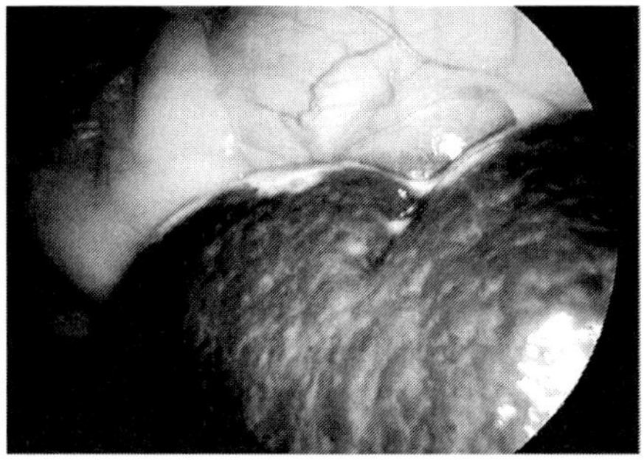
Spleen

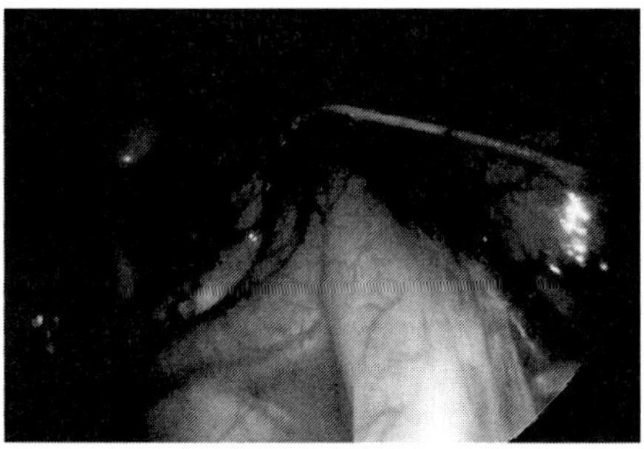
Uterus

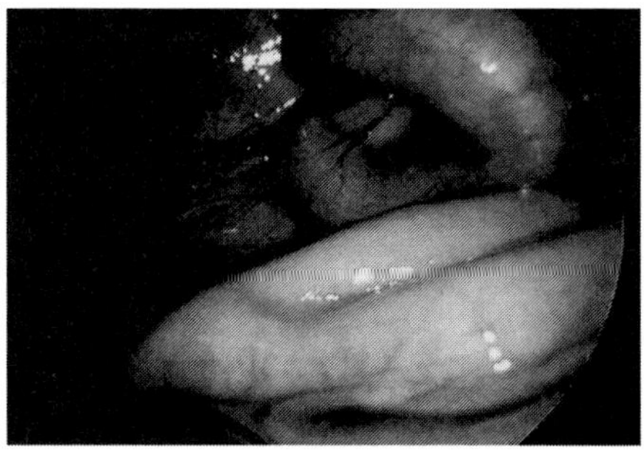
Oviduct

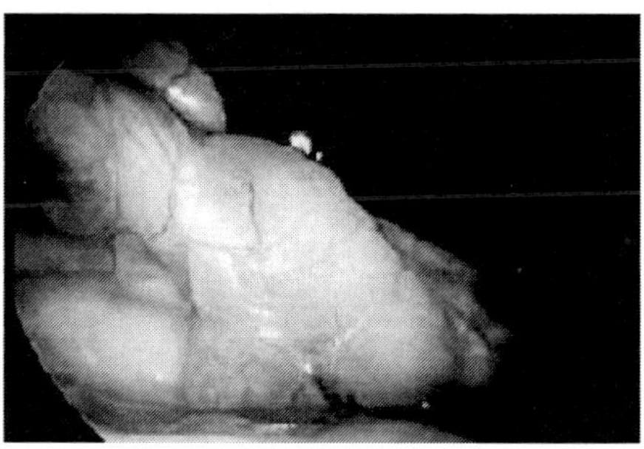
Pancreas

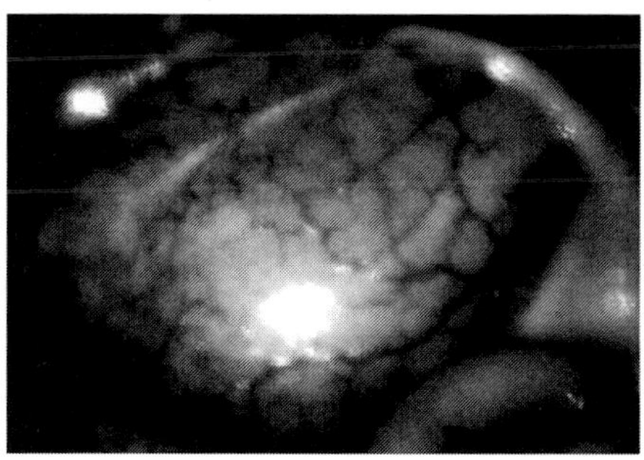
Urinary Bladder

Laparoscopic Diagnosis of different Intraperitoneal lesions

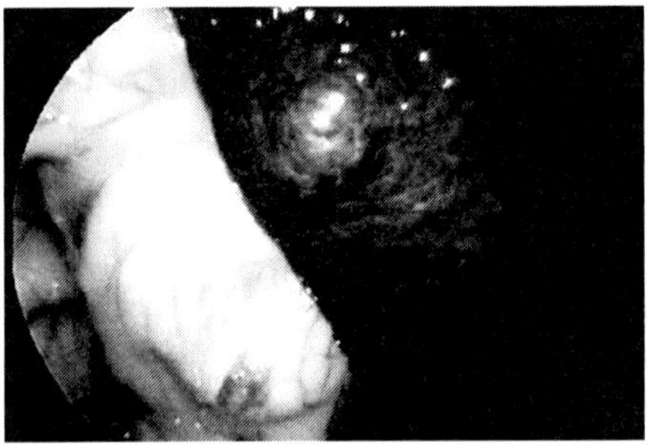

Splenic abscess

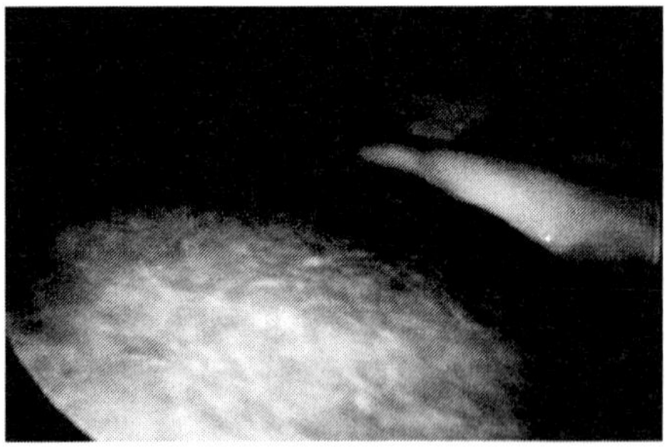

Spleenomegaly

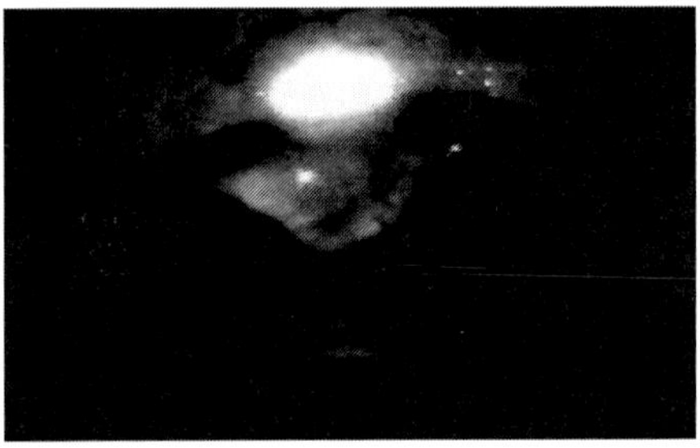

Splenic Wound

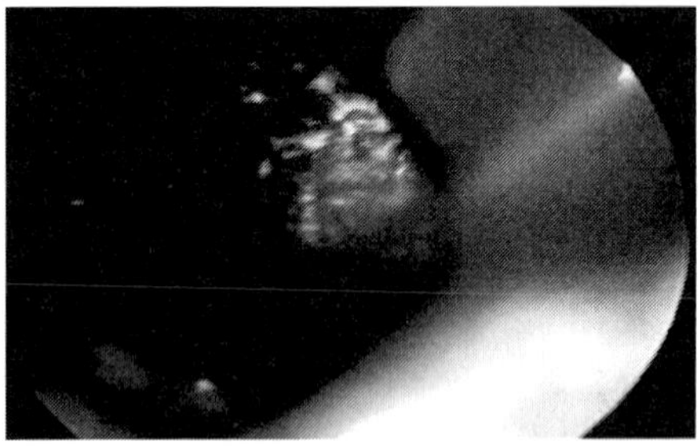

Splenic tumour

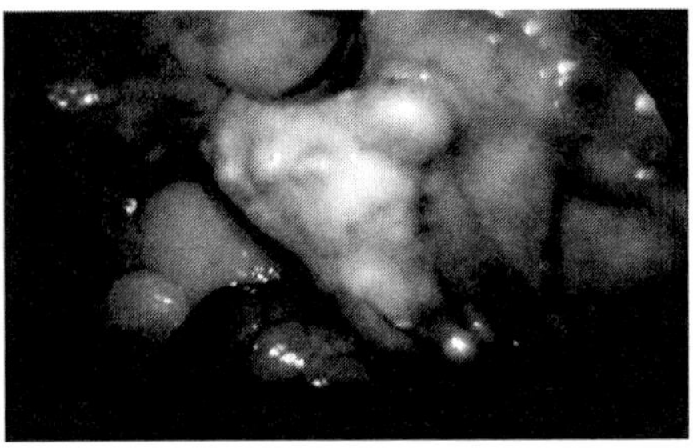

Polycystic ovary

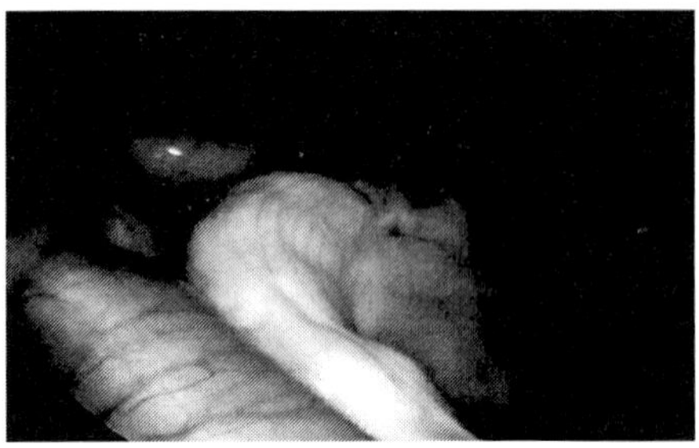

Mummified fetus

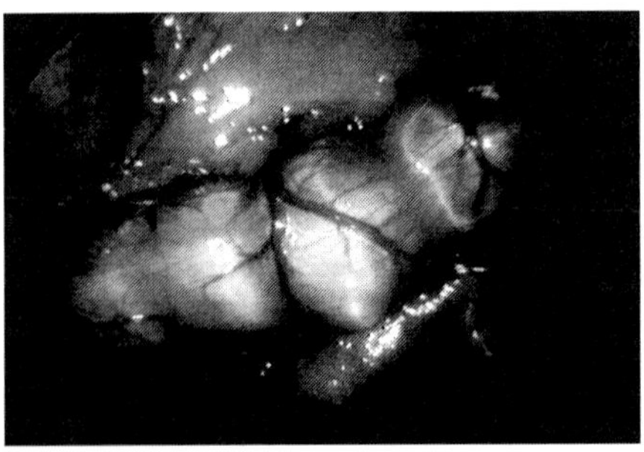

Faecolith

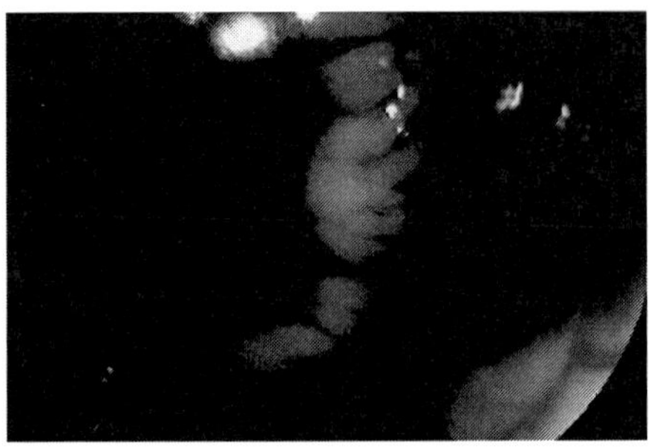

Haemoperitoneum

Laparoscopic diagnosis of intestinal intussusception in dog

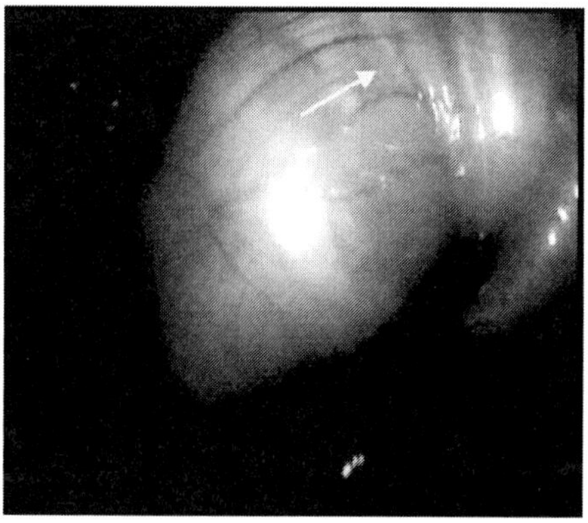

A

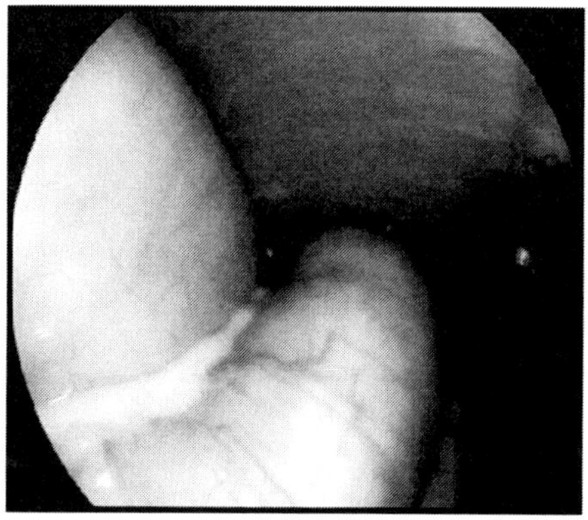

B

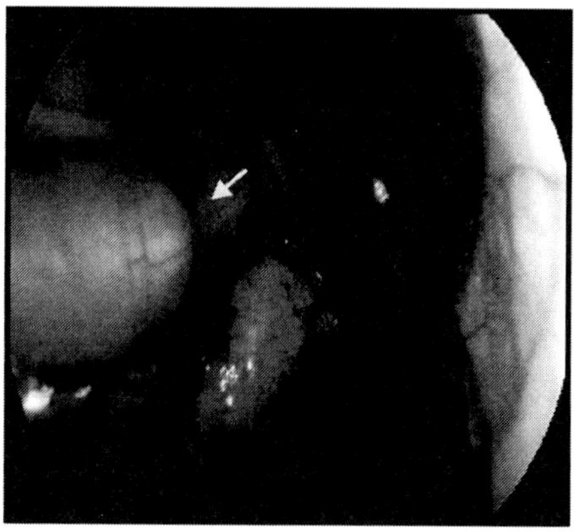

C

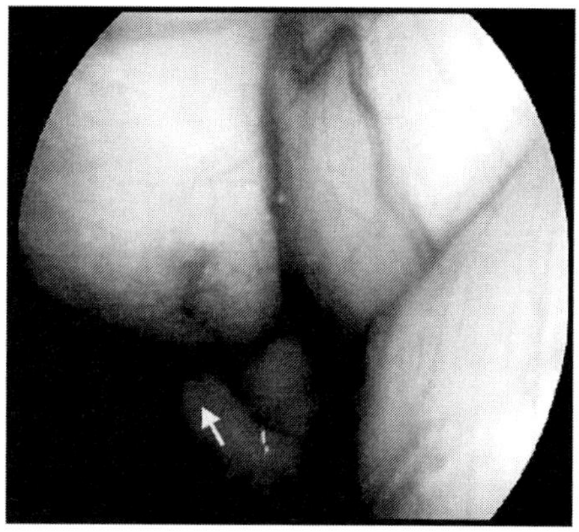

D

❑❑❑

7

Laparoscopic Guided Organ Biopsy and Minor Surgery

Laparoscopy is not only used in the examination of the abdominal cavity organs, surgical treatment but also in the diagnosis of the different disease conditioned by biopsy examination (removal of a sample of tissue from the living body for histopathological examination). Biopsy is indicated to ascertain a correct diagnosis, specific therapy and accurate prognosis. Laparoscopy is becoming an alternative method of monitoring biopsies of internal organs. It permits precise localization and accurate site on the various abdominal organs surface such as kidney, liver, spleen etc. Since, it is relatively noninvasive so it ranks highest amongst biopsy techniques. The technique allows visual control over the biopsy procedure, which considerably limits post biopsy complications and increases the likelihood of obtaining diagnostically useful biopsy specimens.

The different organs from which biopsy sample can be taken through laparoscopy are as follows:

- Liver
- Kidney
- Pancreas
- Gall bladder
- Intestine
- Uterus
- Spleen

- Urinary bladder
- Prostate glands
- Adrenal glands
- Ovarian tissue.

Indications for liver biopsy

- Hepatitis
- Cirrhosis
- Liver carcinoma
- Hepatomegaly
- Unexplained liver-specific biochemistries
- Abnormal liver function tests
- Response to therapy for liver diseases
- Copper hepatotoxicity
- Evaluation of extra hepatic biliary system.

Indications for spleen biopsy

- Spleenomegaly
- Splenic abscess
- Splenic tumour.

Indications for pancreas biopsy

- Pancreatitis
- Primary pancreatic disease
- Chronic fibroid pancreatitis
- Pancreatic neoplasia.

Instrumentation

(a) Instruments and equipments for laparoscopic biopsy

- One 0 or 30° forward oblique, 5 mm telescope.
- One Veres pneumoperitoneum needle of 120 mm length with spring loaded blunt stylet.
- One 5mm spring loaded safety trocars with two cannulae.
- One pair biopsy forceps.
- Electronic, fully automatic carbon dioxide endoflator with high-pressure hose gas connector.
- Halogen/Xenon light source having 250 Watt twin lamps with flexible fiber-optic light cable.
- Digital video camera.
- Medical grade colour monitor.
- Digital video captures system (L-cap) on 3.5 inches floppy disc/ writable CD.
- Combined monopolar and bipolar coagulator (e.g. Megatom 400) for electrocautery.

(b) General surgical instruments in a standard surgical pack

All the laparoscopic instruments should be sterilized in a closed formalin vaporizer chamber for 24 h before surgery. They are soaked in 1.5% chlorhexidin solution for 30 min, rinse with sterile distilled water and wipe with dry sterile gauze.

Preoperative preparation

Animals should be fasted for 12-24 h before laparoscopy and water should be withheld on the morning of the procedure. The urinary bladder, stomach and colon ideally should be empty. Inadvertent puncture of the urinary bladder is possible by the trocar or Veress needle if it is full especially in very small animals.

Preparation of surgical site

The skin over the mid-ventral/lateral abdomen are shaved, cleaned and scrubbed with chlorhexidin solution, wiped with 70% alcohol and painted with povidone iodine.

Anesthesia

Animals should be premedicated with atropine sulphate at the dose rate of 0.04-mg/kg body weight subcutaneously. After 10 minutes, general anaesthesia is achieved with combination of xylazine hydrochloride @ 1.0 mg/kg and ketamine hydrochloride @ 10.0 mg/kg body weight intramuscularly. If required, additional dose of ketamine hydrochloride @ 5 mg/kg and diazepam @ 0.2 mg/ kg body weight intravenously may be administered.

Laparoscopic biopsy of liver

Laparoscopic liver biopsy is considered by many to be a preferred method of obtaining a liver biopsy. Other diagnostic modalities often do not provide sufficient enough information on the liver. Using this approach one is able to examine over 85% of the liver surface, take directed tissue biopsies and monitor for excessive bleeding. The liver is generally evaluated through the right lateral mid-abdominal approach. A significant greater area of liver can be visualized from the right side compared with a ventral or left approach. The right lateral, right medial and caudate lobes of the liver as well as the gall bladder and extra hepatic biliary tract can be thoroughly examined from the right side. A left approach is generally made only if disease involving the left lateral or medial lobe is suspected. Prior to liver biopsy the coagulation parameters are generally evaluated including a bleeding time. Although caogulopathies are a relative contraindication of liver biopsy the coagulation status does not necessarily predict if the patient will bleed from a liver biopsy.

The animal is placed on the operating table in left lateral recumbency. The procedure described in chapter 6 is adopted for laparoscopic examination. A complete examination is undertaken and should proceed in an orderly sequence to examine both the liver and its adjacent structures. The surface of the liver should be examined carefully for any focal or generalized changes. The normal liver should extend caudally to the level of the costal arch and should have a smooth surface with sharp borders. The liver should be of a uniform deep red colour. As the laparoscope is moved close to the liver, the operator will be able to detect the portal areas, as well as a uniform sinusoidal configuration. This is possible as a result of the magnification capabilities of most laparoscopes as they are moved close to the tissue being examined.

Pathological changes of the liver can be detected grossly. Abnormal gross liver changes that can be readily appreciated include hepatic lipidosis (the liver has a pale mustard colour with friable texture), glycogen laden liver, metastatic or multifocal neoplasia (raised and often discolored tumor nodules with central cavitations or depressions are seen), nodular hyperplasia (multiple raised nodules without central depressions and with a yellow fatty appearance), cirrhosis, cholangihepatitis, extra hepatic biliary obstruction etc. liver size and presence of any venous plexuses suggestive of acquired collateral shunting are readily appreciated.

After selection of the biopsy site another 6mm safety trocar and cannula is inserted 4 to 5 cm lateral to the previous site. The laparoscopic biopsy forceps is inserted through the second cannula. With the guidance of the telescope, the biopsy forceps should be advanced to the selected site for liver biopsy. The biopsy forceps is then connected to electrocautery equipment. Cutting of the liver tissue carries out with the biopsy forceps and the site is cauterized with the same forceps. The liver fragment obtained is taken out and transfer into 10% formal saline solution for fixing and later examine for histopathological examination. The same procedure is repeated for obtaining more number of biopsy specimens from liver as desired. The biopsy site should be examined for any hemorrhage. The telescope, CO_2 hosepipe and biopsy forceps are then remove from the trocars and the CO_2 gas from the abdomen is allowed to escape through the sleeve of the cannula. After evacuation of the gas from abdominal cavity, the trocars remove and the skin incision is close with one or two simple interrupted sutures.

A recent study emphasized the benefit of laparoscopic cup biopsies when two 18g needle biopsies were compared to laparoscopic cup biopsies. The needle samples only correlated approximately half the time compared with the larger laparoscopic cup biopsies. Not only is there the advantage of the larger biopsy samples using the oval cup forceps but is the ability to direct the biopsy to a specific area to sample. With this method one is also able to obtain enough tissue for culture or other tissue analysis.

Laparoscopic renal biopsy

Laparoscopy is well studied for the evaluation and biopsy of the kidney. To biopsy the kidney, one can use an automatic "core type" biopsy needle (Vet-Core Biopsy needle, 16g diameter, Cook Veterinary Products). The advantage is the direct visualization of the kidney that allows the operator to navigate the biopsy needle to the desired site to be sampled and also the ability to monitor for excessive postoperative bleeding. Prior to a kidney biopsy an adequate renal evaluation is necessary including renal excretory function, ultrasonography or intravenous urography. This is important to know to help select which kidney to sample. Unless there is specific indications to biopsy the left kidney is preferred because it is less movable. The left kidney biopsy through a left lateral approach is more difficult because of the location of the spleen underlying the usual cannula entry site. Using a right lateral mid- abdominal telescope placement the right kidney is easily visualized. Once the area of the kidney to biopsy is determined a biopsy needle directed to the site. The biopsy needle is seated through the renal capsule and then tissue biopsy is collected followed by needle cauterization. The biopsy needle is then removed from the abdominal cavity. Additional samples are taken if the first sample is not considered to be suitable. During renal biopsy, one should avoid directing the needle deep into the kidney involving the cortico-medullary junction of the kidney where the large arcuate vessels are located.

Laparoscopic intestinal biopsy

Small intestinal biopsies can be obtained using the laparoscope by the technique of grasping and then exteriorizing that portion of intestine through the abdominal wall. The intestinal biopsy samples are then obtained from the exteriorized bowel as would be done through a standard surgical biopsy. The technique involves using a

5 mm atraumatic grasping forceps with multiple teeth to grasp the intestine to be sampled. Once the location is determined the anti-mesenteric boarder if the intestine is firmly grasped with the forceps and the intestine is then pulled to the cannula. A scalpel blade is then used to increase the cannula incision long enough to exteriorize the loop of the bowel. One can watch the scalpel blade internally enter parallel to the cannula shaft and then cut away from the cannula to incision length. Once the cannula incision is extended a 3-4 cm loop of intestine is exteriorized and stay sutures are used in the intestine to prevent it from falling back into the abdominal cavity. A small full thickness biopsy is then obtained in the same manner as one would use when performing an open abdominal surgical biopsy. The intestine is then returned to the abdominal cavity.

The intestinal biopsy should be the last laparoscopic procedure to perform because the pneumoperitoneum is lost during the procedure. Recently, a technique for multiple biopsies of intestine using a serosal patch graft has also been described. This technique involves retaining each segment of bowel biopsied using stay sutures after exteriorization and biopsy and then the different biopsy sites are sutured together to create a serosal patch graft.

Laparoscopic pancreatic biopsy

Laparoscopic forceps can also be used to biopsy the pancreas. The adage "to never touch the pancreas for fear of inducing pancreatitis" does not appear to occur following laparoscopy pancreatic biopsy. It is reported that pancreatic biopsies generally free of complications and a study evaluating laparoscopic pancreatic biopsies in normal dogs found no postoperative complications or indications of secondary pancreatitis. Indications for pancreatic biopsies would include cases suspected of having either acute or chronic pancreatitis or pancreatic neoplasia. Laparoscopy is used by some surgeons to confirm the presence of acute pancreatitis and then to concurrently place a jejunostomy feeding tube for continued patient nutritional management. Chronic pancreatitis is also a common finding in the cats either alone or in conjunction with liver diseases and laparoscopy is the best means for diagnosis for this condition. Punch type biopsy forceps work well for pancreatic biopsies, however, the cup biopsy forceps can also be used as well. To obtain pancreatic biopsy, the right lateral approach is preferred. This approach gives an excellent view of the duodenum, the right limb of the pancreas as well as the extrahepatic biliary system and liver. The biopsy site selected should be at the edge of the pancreas away from the location of the pancreatic ducts that will traverse the center of the gland and subsequently enter the duodenum with the common bile duct. It is advisable to take only one or two representative biopsy sample of the pancreas unless multiple lesions are present.

Other laparoscopic biopsy techniques

A number of other biopsy techniques can also be performed with laparoscopic direction. This includes biopsy of mass lesions, lymph nodes, spleen and adrenal gland. Splenic biopsies are generally safe to perform using the cup type biopsy forceps or a biopsy needle. The technique, precautions and coagulation control methods are the same to liver biopsy method. Adrenal biopsies are sometimes performed when an adrenal mass is identified. Care should be taken because bleeding followed adrenal biopsy is common and haemostatic precautions are usually necessary. Cup forceps are used to obtain adrenal biopsy. Laparoscopy may also be used to determine the cause of unexplained abdominal effusion. The fluid is aspirated under endoscopic direction to enable examination of the abdominal content.

There are a number of minimally invasive surgical procedures that can be performed by using laparoscopy.

Feeding tube placement

Duodenostomy or jejunostomy feeding tube can be placed using the laparoscope simply by exteriorizing a respective piece of intestine through the abdominal wall and inserting the tube externally. The technique of bowel exteriorization is similar to that described for intestinal biopsy. The intestine must be pexied to the abdominal wall in conjunction with the tube placement. A gastrostomy feeding tube can also be placed using the laparoscopy by simply by exteriorizing the body of the stomach through the left abdominal wall and then inserting the tube externally following a gatropexy.

Cryptorchid surgery

A testicle that is located in the abdominal cavity can be removed easily using laparoscopy. The dog is placed in dorsal recumbency with the table tilted with the head in the lower position. Internal inguinal rings are inspected to determine the presence of vas deference and testicular arteries. An absence of these structures in the inguinal canal means the testicle is ectopic. The ectopic testicle is usually readily visible upon entering the abdominal cavity. The vascular pedicle and vas deference are ligated with either pre-tied suture or endoclip. The ectopic testicle is transected and removed through the cannula hole outside.

Laparoscopic Cystoscopy

It is also possible to examine the lumen of the urinary bladder using a laparoscopy technique. The bladder of the most female dogs can easily be evaluated using rigid transurethral cystoscopy that precludes the need for laparoscopic evaluation. However, in male dog, it is most difficult to evaluate because of their urethral anatomy.

Gastric foreign body removal

Gastric foreign bodies that cannot be removed with gastroscopy can be accessed for removal with this laparoscopy technique. In this method the body of the stomach exteriorized similar to gastrostomy tube placement. Stay sutures are placed from the stomach wall to the skin to prevent the stomach from falling back into the abdominal cavity. A gastrotomy incision is performed of sufficient size for removal of the foreign materials. Gastric contents are aspirated and gastric lavage can be performed, if indicated. The telescope can then be introduced directly into the stomach for examination of the contents and for removal of foreign material.

Laparoscopic liver biopsy through cauterization in small animal

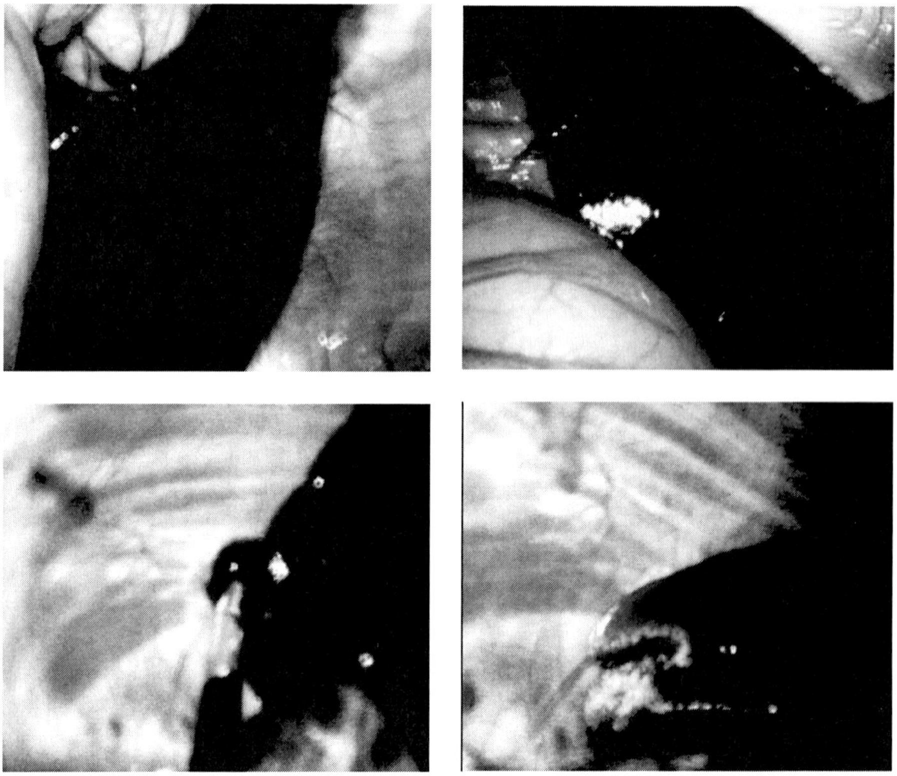

Dog

Laparoscopic liver biopsy through cauterization in small animal

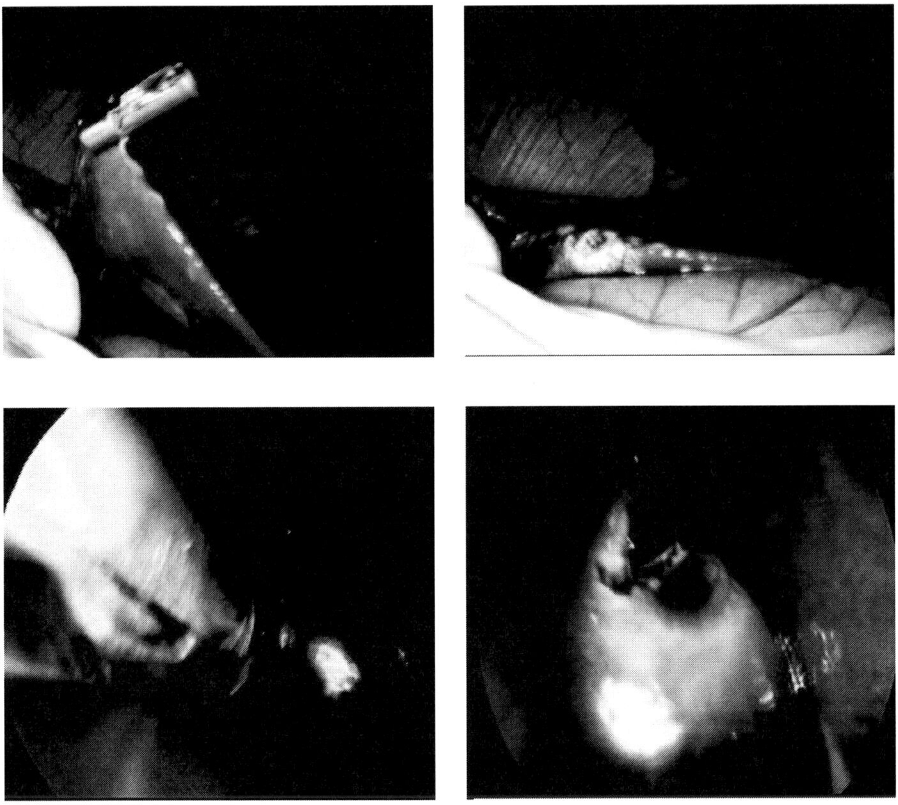

Goat

Laparoscopic Liver Biopsy through Cauterization in Small Animal

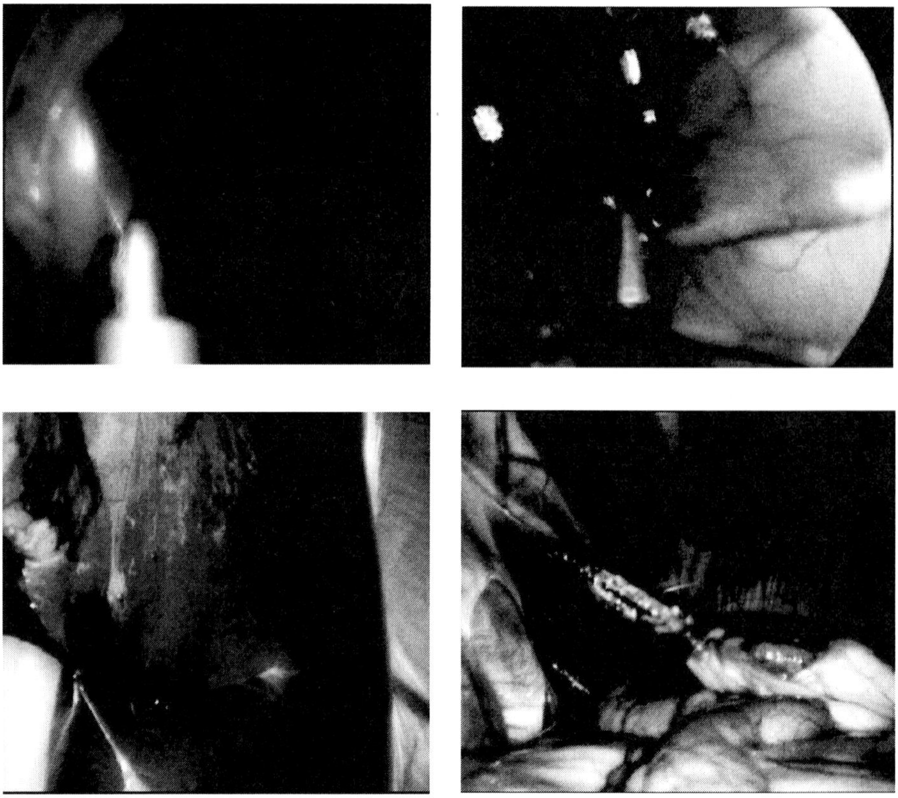

Rabbit

Laparoscopic biopsy of liver and gall bladder

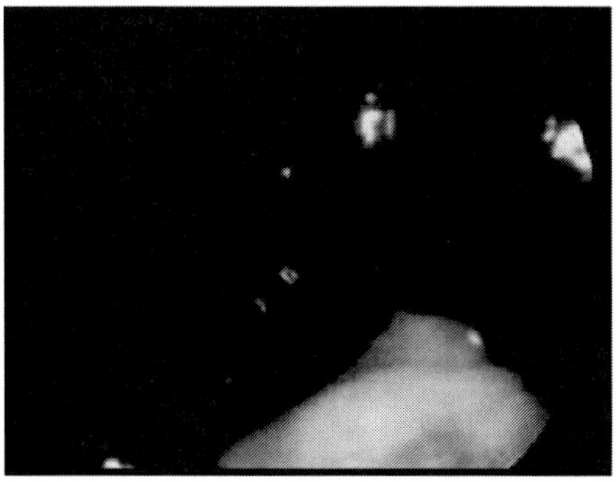

Laparoscopic visualization of liver surface

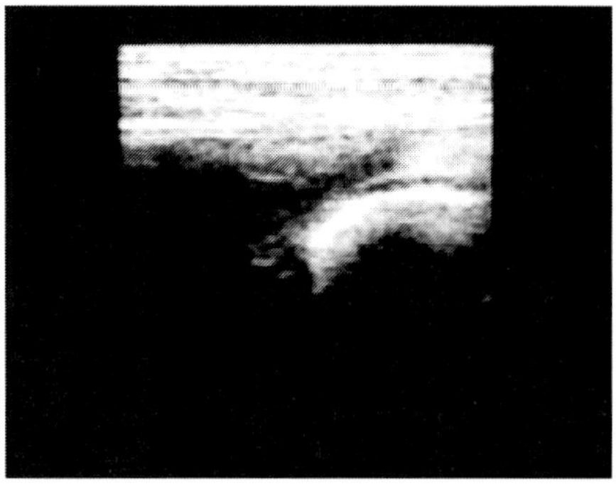

Visualization of liver by ultrasonography

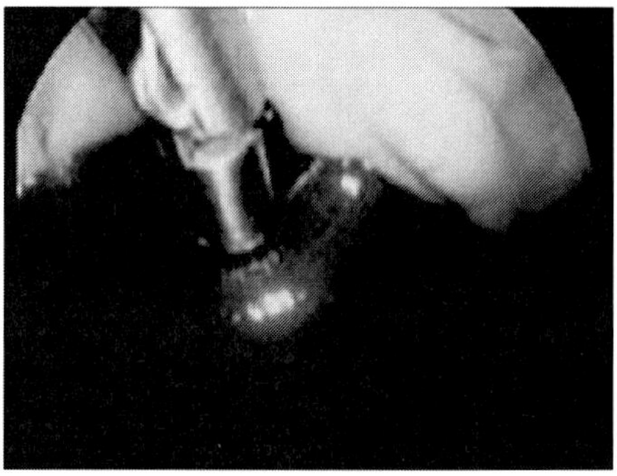

Liver biopsy using biopsy forceps under laparoscopic guidance

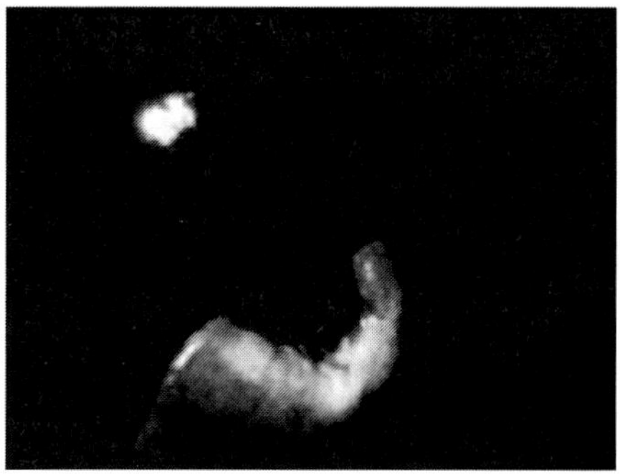

Biopsy site just after laparoscopic biopsy

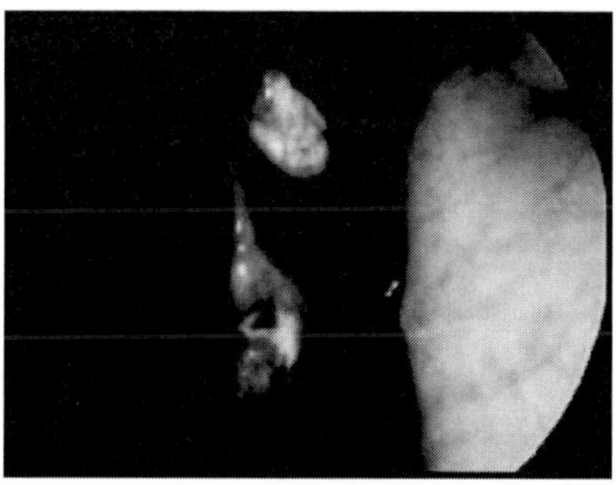

Biopsy site after 7 days of laparoscopic biopsy

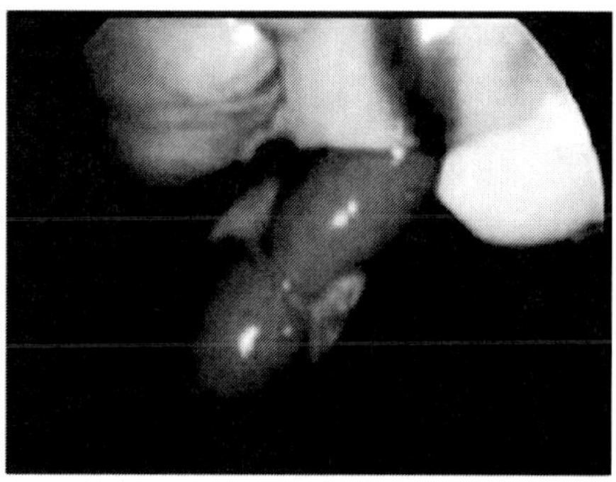

Biopsy site after 15 days of laparoscopic biopsy

Laparoscopic diagnosis of different liver diseases

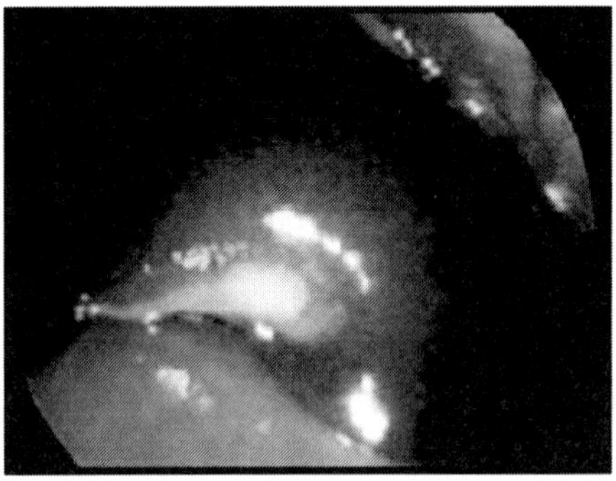

Biopsy site after 30 days of laparoscopic biopsy

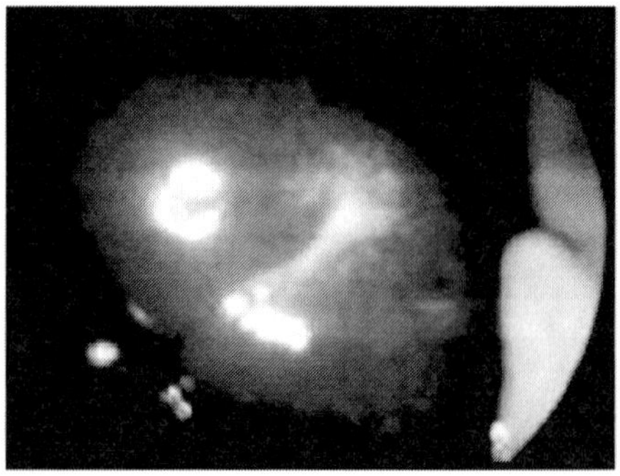

Biopsy site after 60 days of laparoscopic biopsy

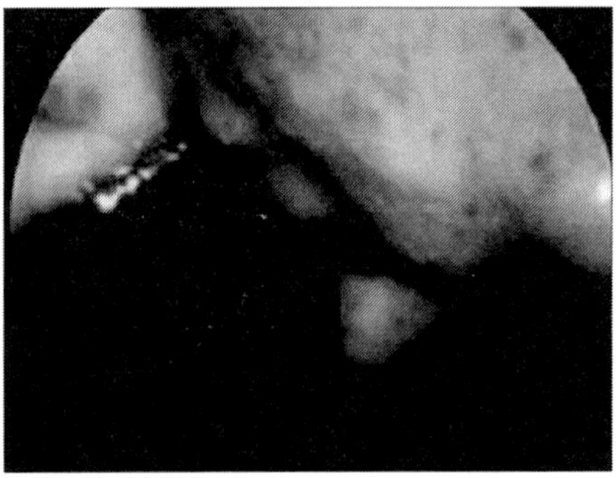

Laparoscopic visualization liposarcoma of liver

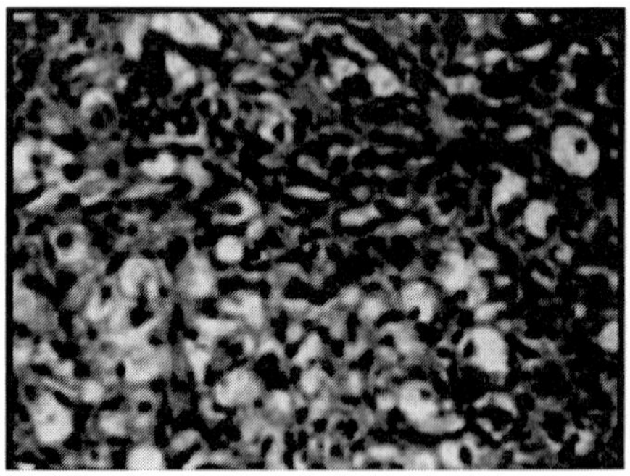

Liposarcoma of liver-tumourous adepocytes lined by hyperchromatic nuclei (H&Ex260)

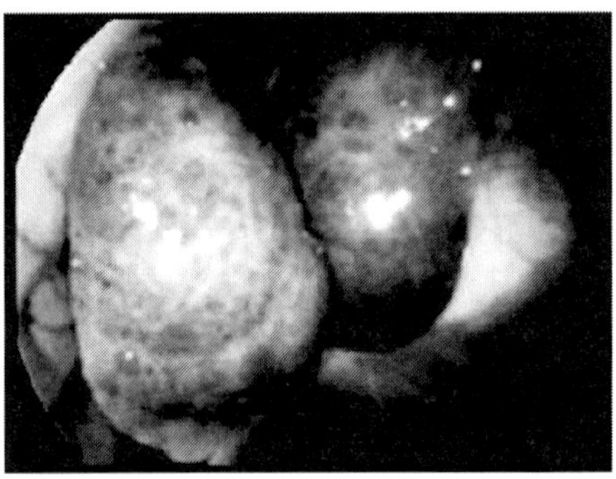

Laparoscopic visualization of liver having cirrhosis

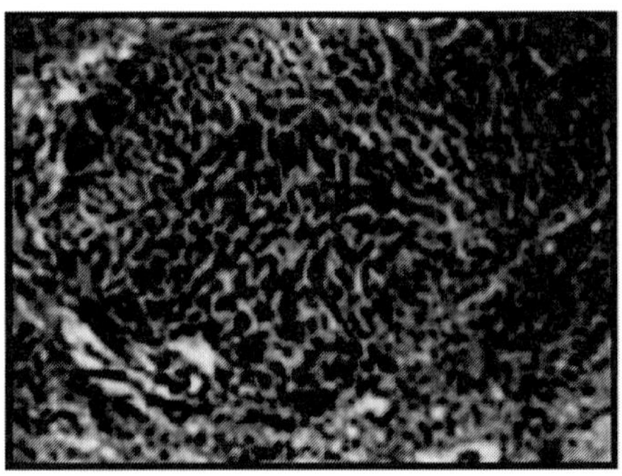

Cirrhosis-hepatocytes surrounded by fibrous connective tissue (H&Ex100)

Laparoscopic diagnosis of different liver diseases

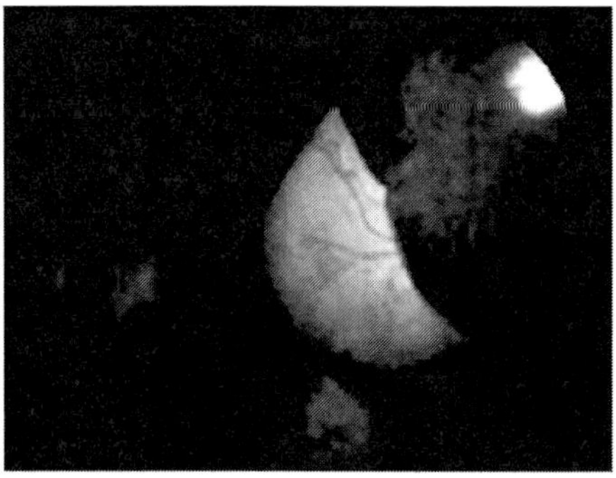

Laparoscopic visualization of hepatitis

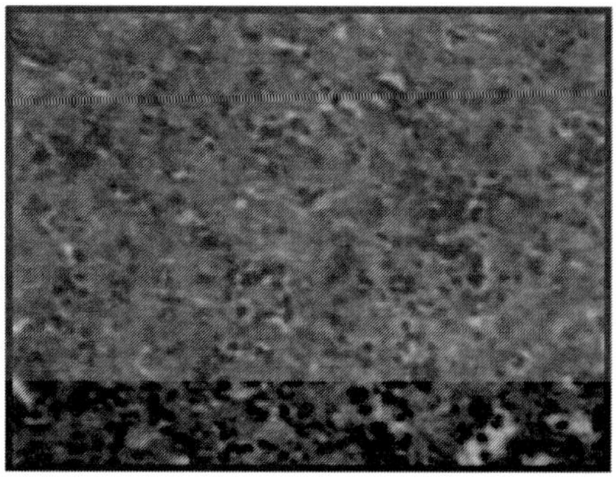

Hepatitis-swollen hepatocytes with large vesicular nuclei and Sinusoids filled with leucocytes (H&E X 260)

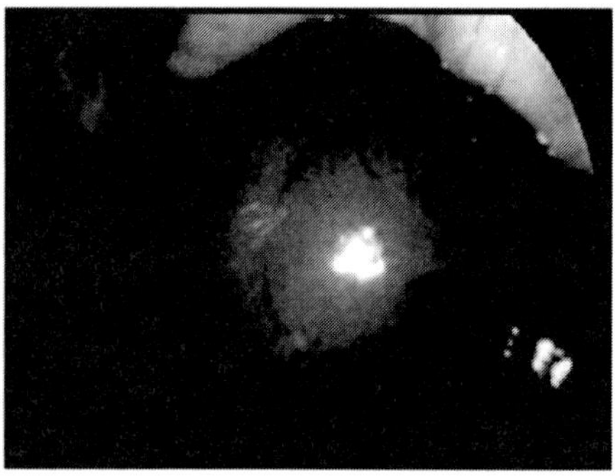

Laparoscopic visualization of hepatomegaly

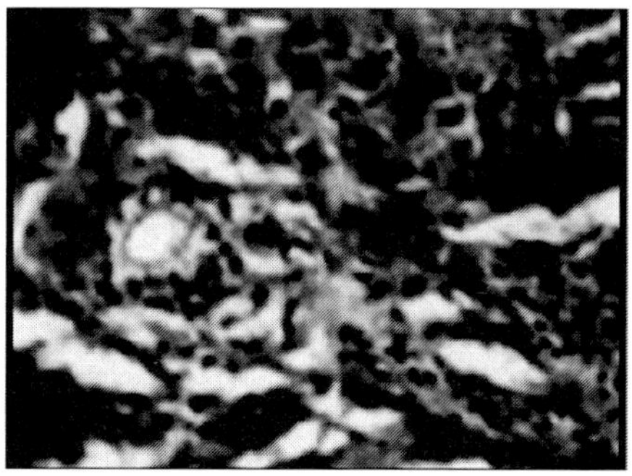

Distended portal area with vacuolated bile duct epithelial cells (H&E X 330)

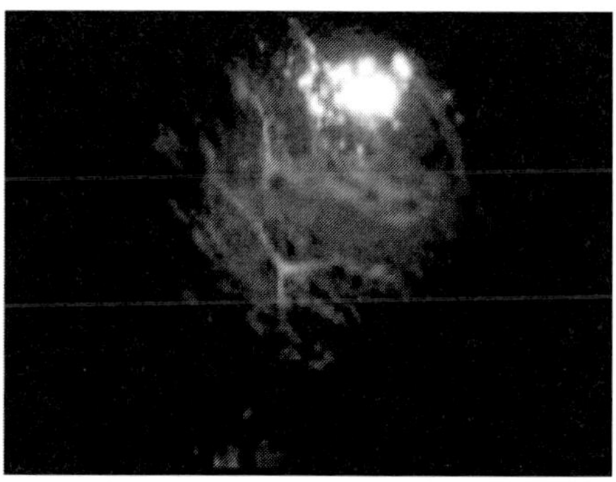

Laparoscopic visualization of liver surface showing bridging fibrosis

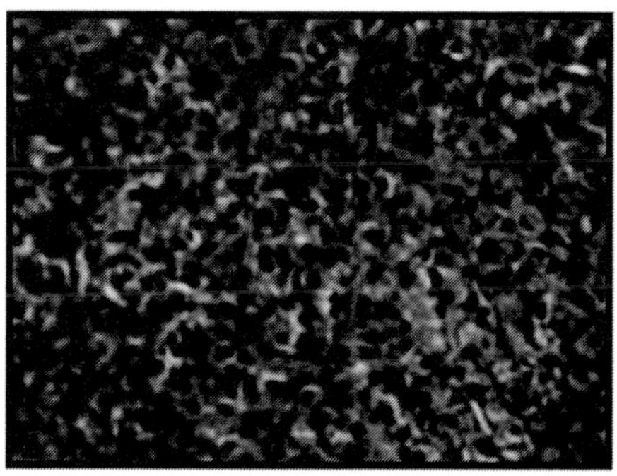

Hepatic parenchyma in dog with bridging fibrosis of liver (H&E X 200)

8

Laparoscopic Ancillary Diagnostic Procedures

The most common indication for laparoscopy is to examine and biopsy the abdominal organs or masses. Additional diagnostic procedures that can be performed using laparoscopic guidance include gall bladder puncture to collect bile, contrast radiographic techniques for the diagnosis of bile duct obstructions, overdistension of gall bladder, portography and splenic pulp pressure measurement.

Laparoscopic ancillary diagnostic procedures

- Biliary evaluation
- Cholecystocentesis
- Cholecystography
- Cholecystocholangiography
- Splenic pulp pressure measurement
- Splenoportography

Instrumentation

(a) Equipments for laparoscopic ancillary diagnostic procedures

- As mentioned in chapter 7.

(b) Instruments for laparoscopic ancillary diagnostic procedures

- 20 G and 10cm long spinal needle/ biopsy needle

- Syringes (5 and 10 ml) for aspiration of bile and injection of contrast agent.

(c) General surgical instruments in a standard surgical pack

Contrast media

- Iohexol' (300 mg/ml)
- Meglumine iodipamide.

The biopsy needle and other surgical instruments are sterilized by autoclaving at 121^{0}C for 30 minutes under 15 lbs. pressure.

The preoperative preparation of animal and anaesthesia has been described in chapter 7.

Biliary evaluation / Cholecystocentesis

A right side approach is used to evaluate the gallbladder, extra hepatic ducts and common bile ducts. The procedure for laparoscopic examination has already been described in chapter 7. After identification of the liver and different lobes is identified, the surface of the organ is carefully examined. The CO_2 pressure is slowly increased until the gall bladder is fully visualized between the quadrate and right medial lobes of the liver. Slight adjustments in the position of the animal are to be made for clear visualization of gall bladder. The right lateral lobe of the liver is elevated to observe the hilium of the liver, the gall bladder and the remainder of the biliary system. The normal gall bladder, when palpated, should be soft and fluctuant and the ductal system should not be distended. After a complete evaluation of the extra hepatic biliary system and adjacent structures, aspiration of bile from the gall bladder can be performed. One 20gauge and 10cm spinal needle is satisfactory for this procedure and it is inserted into the abdominal cavity at a site on right abdomen (3-5 cm lateral to midline) below the right costal arch. Under the guidance of telescope, the spinal needle is then direct between lobes of the liver until it reaches near the surface of the gall bladder. An area on the gall bladder devoid of blood vessels should be select and the spinal needle is inserted into the gall bladder by piercing its wall slowly taking care not to tear it. After inserting the needle into the sac, the stylet of the spinal needle is carefully removed and its hub is connected to a 10ml sterile syringe. The bile is aspirated into the syringe as much as possible from the decompressed gall bladder to prevent leakage when the needle is removed. The bile should be submitted for colour, consistency, cytological examination, bacterial culture and sensitivity and other biliary evaluation.

There are two precautions one should take when doing this procedure. First, it is important to assure the needle is placed through the abdominal wall caudal to the diaphragm for fear of producing a Pneumothorax and that is important to decompress the gall bladder as much as possible to prevent leakage.

Cholecystography and Cholecystocholangiography

A contrast study can be performed under laparoscopic guidance in animals suspected for extra hepatic bile duct obstruction. After collection of bile 5-10 ml of sterile radiographic contrast agent Meglumine iodipamide (e.g. iohexol) as per body weight is injected into the gall bladder directly through the same needle. The volume of contrast media to be injected in to the gall bladder should be adjusted to prevent gall bladder from over distension. Over distension may result in leakage of the contrast agent. After injecting the contrast media the spinal needle is carefully removed from the gall bladder followed by telescope and cannula. If the biliary tract is patent, contrast material should easily be passed into the duodenum. Serial radiographs at different intervals are necessary for visualization of this passage, detection of any abnormality and to check the patency of the bile duct. The contrast will generally remain within the biliary system long enough to perform the radiographic studies. After the anesthetic revival, the animal is fed with a high fat diet and allowed to walk to get some exercise to facilitate the emptying of the gall bladder.

Laparoscopy-guided cholecystography is superior to routine intravenous cholecystography owing to the safety, gall bladder contrast and the added facility of bile collection for evaluation through the same needle used for injection of contrast agent into gall bladder. Moreover, the laparoscopic technique is added some advantages like detection of any rupture of the gall bladder, leakage of bile, presence of any adhesions of the gall bladder and absence of increased risk of possible hypersensitivity to the contrast agent given intravenously.

Splenic pulp pressure

This technique is performed to demonstrate portal hypertension secondary to liver disease and it can be performed under laparoscopic guidance and visualization. To perform this procedure, the animal should be approached from a left mid abdominal approach. Precaution should be taken to avoid excessive splenic trauma. After proper visualization of spleen and evaluation a 20 gauge and 10cm spinal needle is inserted through the ventrolateral abdominal wall near the area of spleen. The needle should direct in such a manner that it will traverse the spleen parallel with the long axis. Under laparoscopic visualization, the needle is inserted 1-3 cm into the center of the splenic parenchyma. Once the needle is seated firmly within the spleen, the laparoscope is removed and the insufflated CO_2 gas is evacuated before pressure recording are performed. Splenic pulp pressure is generally measured in centimeters of water (normal: 10-15 cm of water) using a simple manometer. After pressure recording, the needle is removed and spleen is again checked for any hemorrhage. In chronic liver diseases and cirrhosis, the pressure may be high up to 30 to 40 cm of water.

Instrumentation for laparoscopic biopsy and ancillary procedures

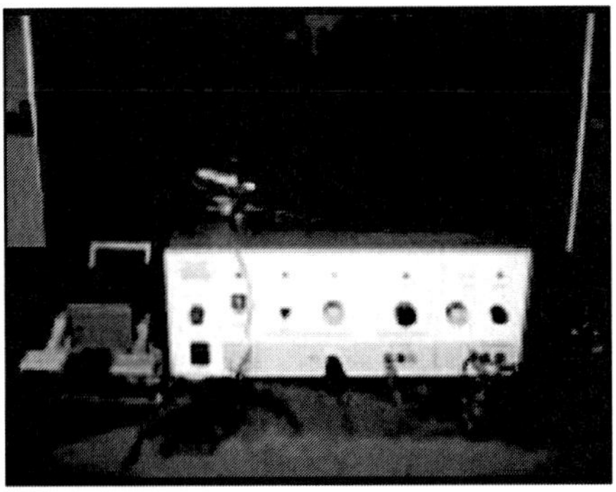

Electro-cautery device
(Megatom 400)

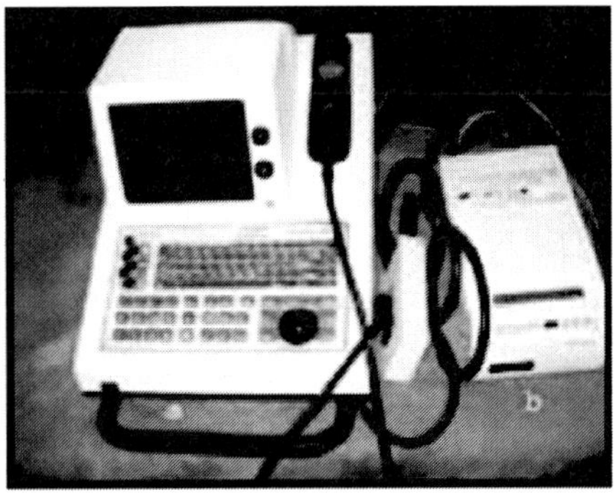

Ultrasonography equipment
a) Monitor, b) Thermoprinter
c) Transducer

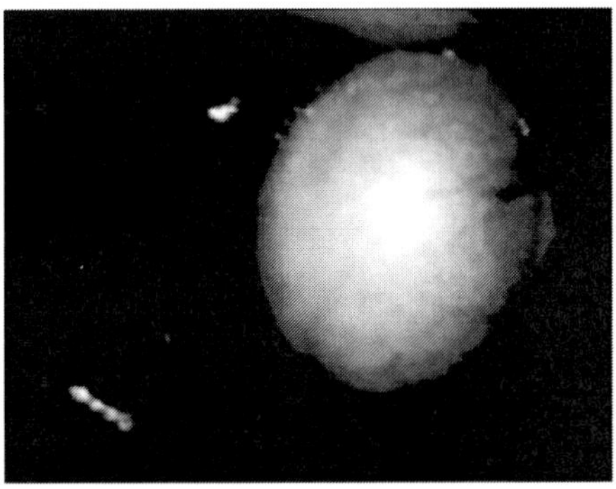

Laparoscopic visualization of gall bladder

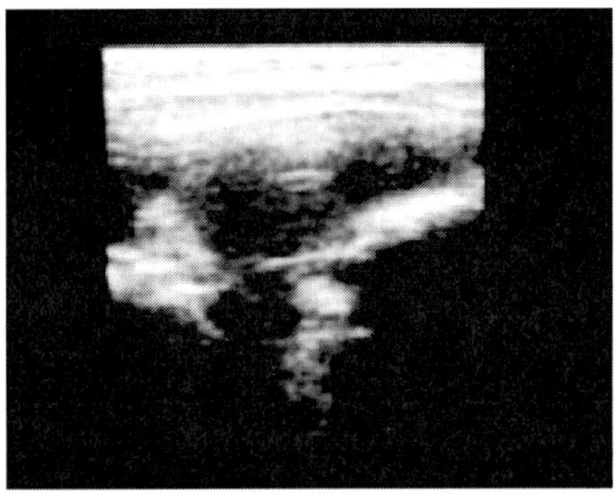

Liver biopsy using percutaneous biopsy needle under ultrasound guidance

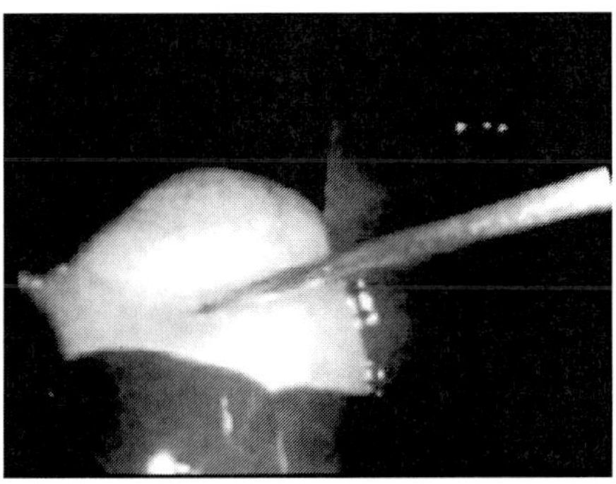

Insertion of spinal needle into gall bladder under laparoscopic guidance

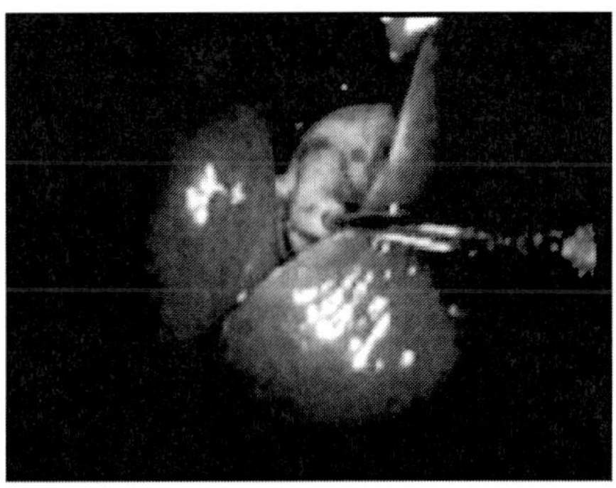

Decompression of gall bladder after aspiration of bile

Laparoscopic Guided Cholecystography

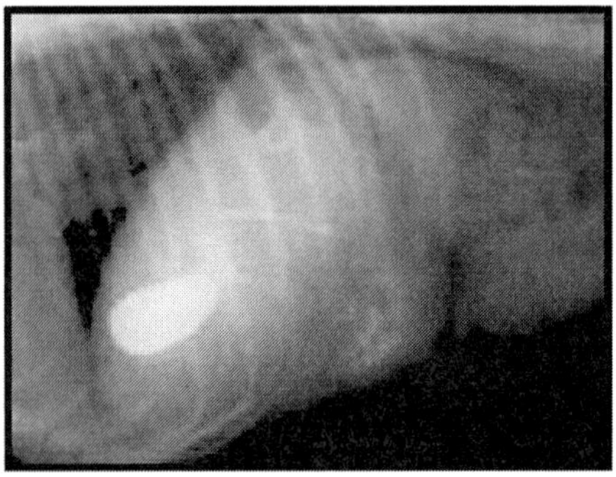

Radiograph taken just after laparoscopy-guided injection of iohexol into Gall bladder

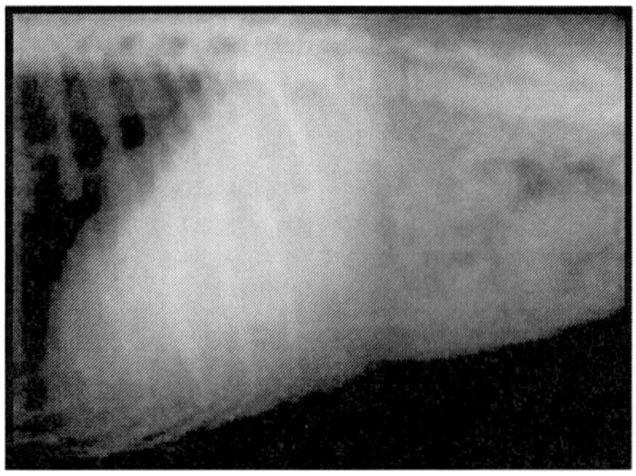

Radiograph taken after 6 hours of a fatty diet following laparoscopic guided Cholecystography

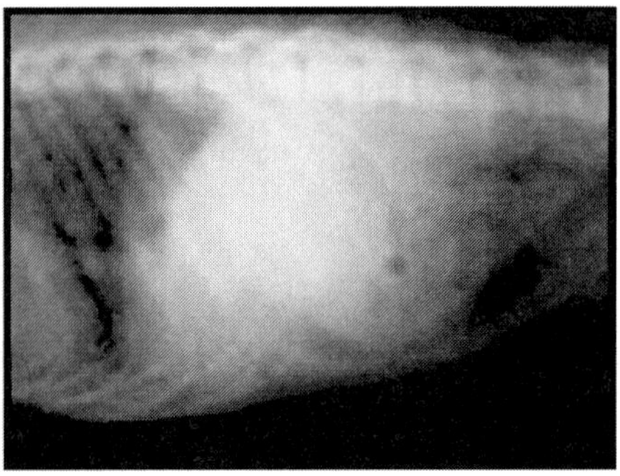

Radiograph taken just after intravenous Cholecystography

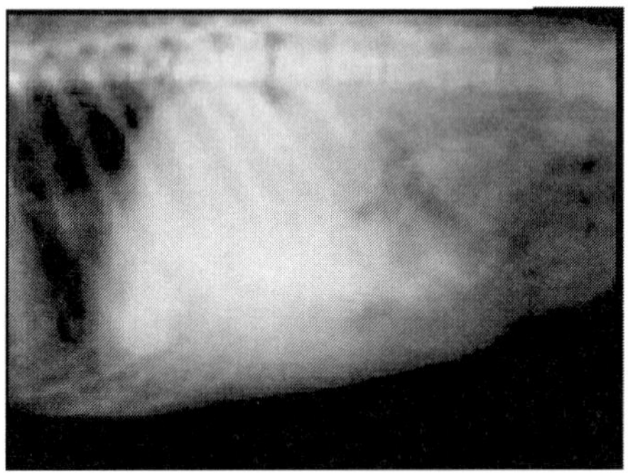

Radiograph taken after 3 hours of intravenous Cholecystography

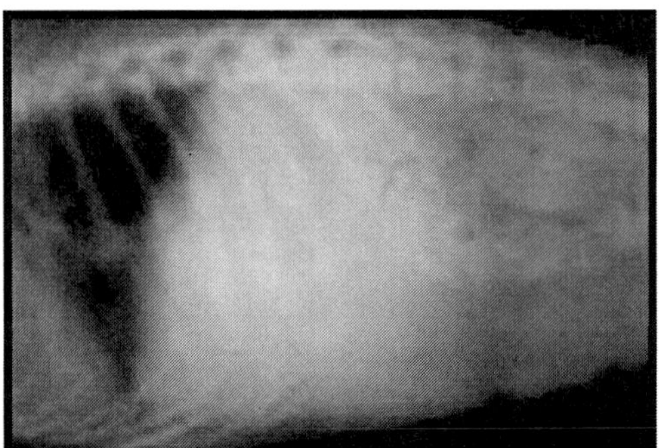

Radiograph taken after 6 hours of a fatty diet following intravenous Cholecystography

Splenoportography

This technique is generally performed to demonstrate portal blood flow and it can be done under laparoscopic guidance and visualization. With this technique it is possible to detect most all congenital or acquired vascular anomalies. The advantage of this technique is that portography can be performed in conjunction with a liver biopsy. Splenoportography involves placement of iodine radiographic contrast into the portal vascular system to outline portal blood flow cranial to where the splenic vein enters the portal vein. It should be performed in X-ray room and on X-ray table. To perform this procedure, the animal should be approached from a left mid-abdominal approach. Establishment of capnoperitoneum and techniques for insertion of laparoscope and spinal needle in to the spleen are similar as described earlier (chapter 7). Once the needle has been placed firmly into the spleen, an intravenous radio opaque iodine contrast agent is injected. A dose of 0.25 to 0.5ml/kg of the contrast agent is injected at the rate of 1-2 ml/ second. Series of radiographs are taken immediately after injection of the contrast agent to demonstrate the pattern of portal blood flow. In most situations one is able to delineate the location of the portal blood flow and can document either a congenital or acquired shunt. It is reported that this procedure is safe and associated with minimal complications.

An alternative method for portography involves exteriorizing jejunal vein for direct catheter placement in a vein. The method of jejunal vein presentation is similar to that used for the intestinal biopsy technique.

Postoperative care

The surgical wound/trocar points should be regularly dressed in animals using povidone iodine and antiseptic cream until healing. Broad-spectrum antibiotic and analgesic should be given to animals that underwent ancillary procedures for 3-5 days. Animal behavior and all vital parameters should be monitored regularly for at least one week post biopsy.

Complications

Following complications can be observed during laparoscopic ancillary diagnostic procedure.

- Anesthetic complications.
- Air embolism.
- Pneumothorax.
- Diaphragm puncture.
- Organ perforation.
- Infection.
- Gall bladder perforation.
- Bile discharge.
- Excessive splenic injury.
- Splenic bleeding.
- Over distension of abdomen.
- Cardio-pulmonary arrest.
- Instrumentation.
- Electro caution during cauterization.

❏❏❏

9

Laparoscopic Sterilization in Bitches

Among the various modern surgical methods, laparoscopy is now held as one of the most potent and promising aids for both diagnostic (laparoscopy) and therapeutic (laparoscopic surgery) use. Laparoscopy is an endoscopic procedure that bridges the gap between clinical evaluation and surgical exploration. The laparoscopic surgical techniques in both and human and veterinary medicine have grown tremendously. Laparoscopy requires a minor surgical intervention and it provides the only available practical means of making repeated direct observation of abdominal viscera. The advantage of surgical laparoscopy over the conventional open surgical laparotomy include faster patient recovery because of smaller surgical sites, decreased hospitalization, improved cosmetic, improved visualization of abdominal organs, lower postoperative morbidity with lower infection rates, and less postoperative pain and stress. Surgeons are commonly looking for more progressive and stressful surgical methods of sterilization in dogs, particularly in canine birth control programs in urban industrial areas. Demographically dense urban and industrial areas require effective animal birth control programs that can overcome the problems of hospitalization, postoperative complications and reduction in the overall cost of operation. In a large scale animal birth control program, the conventional methods of sterilization require a long period between capture of dogs and their release, due to the time taken for the surgical wounds to heal. In this aspect, keyhole surgery (laparoscopic surgery) can revolutionize the entire program, as it needs only a very small surgical wound, which usually needs no postoperative care or regular dressings.

Laparoscopic ovariohysterectomy

Anatomically, the ovaries are approximately 1-3 cm in length and are located along the dorsolateral wall of the abdomen, just distal to the caudal pole of the kidney. The mesovarium and mesometrium attach the ovary and uterine body to the body wall. The suspensory ligament runs to the level of the 13th rib from the cranial pole of the ovary. The ovarian blood supply is via the ovarian artery, a direct branch of the aorta. The left ovarian vein empties into the left renal vein, while the right ovarian vein empties directly into the caudal vena cava. The ovarian artery and veins, as well as the uterine artery and vein, a branch of the internal pudendal artery/vein supply the uterine body and horns.

Numerous uterine diseases have been reported in dogs and cats. This is one reason why elective ovariohysterectomy (OVH) procedures have been recommended for non breeding animals. Follicular cysts have been reported in 16% of dogs and can result in prolonged estrus, cystic mammary hyperplasia and genital fibroleiomyomas. Ovarian and uterine neoplasia is uncommon in dogs, and account for 0.4-1.2 % of canine neoplasms. One of the most serious and potentially life threatening diseases of the female dog is pyometra. Pyometra is a result of cystic endometrial hyperplasia, which is caused by exogenous progesterone secretion. The end result of this disease is a pus filled, infected uterus, glomerulonephritis, and possible septicemia. The pyometra complex is preventable with ovariohysterectomy procedures. OVH has also been shown to reduce the incidence of mammary cancer in dogs. Dogs that underwent ovariohysterectomy prior to their first heat cycle decreased the incidence of mammary tumors to less than 0.5% versus 26% incidence after two heat cycles.

Traditional ovariohysterectomy has been associated with numerous complications. Hemorrhage is one of the commonly occurred complications. Erosion of the vessels occluded by ligatures has been reported 7-16 days postoperatively. Uterine stump pyometra and recurrent estrus can be the result of poor visualization of ovarian tissue and incomplete removal of ovarian tissue. Fistulous tracts have been reported to be the result of an inflammatory reaction to the suture material. These tracts usually form in the flank region due to non absorbable suture material (eg. silk or nylon). Incisional dehiscence is a risk in any celiotomy procedure and may result in herniation of abdominal viscera.

Pain associated with traditional celiotomy is a growing concern for this common elective procedure. Much research has been directed at studying the effects of pain in animals treated by traditional ovariohysterectomy. It is well documented that traditional ovariohysterectomy procedures inflict pain and morbidity in veterinary patients as a result of tissue trauma, organ manipulation, and inflammation. Pet owners have become increasingly concerned about postoperative pain and morbidity associated with open abdominal procedures. The result of these concerns has lead to an increased demand for minimally invasive surgical techniques from the public/ pet owners. Minimally invasive surgical techniques have generated attention in veterinary medicine; just as increased awareness of patient pain control has emerged to the forefront of veterinary research.

The authors are experienced that laparoscopic ovariectomy performed with bipolar cautery decreased ovariectomy operative time, decreased postoperative hemorrhage and easy exteriorization of the ovaries. A second, more recent study, demonstrated decreased pain in laparoscopic ovariohysterectomy procedure, in which the ovarian pedicle ligation were performed with intracorporeal wire ligatures and bipolar cautery. A third study, reported the technique of laparoscopic OVH in 9 dogs treated with the harmonic scalpel. Recently, Robert B. Hancock (2005) compared postoperative pain following ovariohysterectomy via harmonic scalpel assisted laparoscopy (HALO) versus traditional OVH in dogs and concluded that dogs appeared to be less painful with the HALO procedure than traditional OVH. The harmonic scalpel coagulated ovarian and uterine vessels completely with minimal collateral damage to surrounding tissues. The harmonic scalpel-assisted laparoscopic ovariohysterectomy is also a safe alternative to traditional OVH and offers a minimally invasive and less painful surgical procedure.

Instrumentation

A. Laparoscopic instruments

- Telescope 0 or 30^0 forward, oblique, 5 mm telescope.
- Veress needle of 120 mm working length with spring loaded blunt stylet.
- One 5 mm spring loaded safety trocar with two cannulae.
- One 10 mm pyramidal tip trocar with two 11 mm cannulae.
- One pair fenestered grasping forceps.
- One pair of dissecting and grasping forceps.
- One pair of Metzenbaum curve scissors.
- Two adaptors.
- One 10 mm clip applicator.
- Medium sized titanium endoclips.

B. Laparoscopic equipments

- Electronic, fully automatic CO_2 endoflator with high pressure hose CO_2 gas connector, main cord and silicon tubing set, with CO_2 gas cylinder.
- Xenon or halogen light source having 250 Watt twin lamps of 240 VAC power supply with flexible 5-8 mm fibre optic light cable.
- Digital video camera.
- Medical grade colour monitor.
- Digital video capture system with 3.5 inches floppy disc or compact disc.
- Combined unipolar and bipolar coagulator.

C. General surgical instruments

- A standard general surgical pack containing common surgical instruments.

Surgical procedure

After proper anaesthesia, the animal should be placed in dorsal recumbency. Four-quarter drapes are placed approximately 2cm lateral to each row to mammary teats at the xyphoid and the pubis. The animal is then placed in a Trendelenburg position to facilitate cranial displacement of the visceral contents. A small 1cm skin incision is made at umbilicus. One hand grasping the skin around the skin incision and simultaneous insertion of Veress needle by other hand is performed. The underlying structures are palpated before insertion of the needle. Intraperitoneal placement is confirmed by injecting 5 ml of saline through the needle. The solution should flow without resistance and should not return when trying to aspirate. Carbon dioxide insufflation at a rate of 2 L/min with 12 mm Hg pressure gradient is made after connecting the CO_2 gas hose from the endoflator to the luer-lock of Veress needle and then moderate pneumoperitoneum is established. Respiration and capillary perfusion is closely monitored to check over distension. After attaining a sufficient pneumoperitoneum, Veress needle is removed and a 6 mm safety trocar and cannula are inserted into the peritoneum through the Veress needle incision. The trocar is then removed and the gas hose from Veress needle is attached to the cannula. A rigid type telescope connected with the light source (xenon/halogen lamp) and digital camera is then introduced through cannula. The telescope placed through the umbilical port is used to identify the epigastric blood vessels in order to facilitate placement of the paramedian instrument ports under camera supervision. These ports are creating 1cm lateral to the mammary teat in the caudal abdomen, being sure to avoid the caudal superficial epigastric artery. Ports are created by 10mm pyramidal tip trocar and cannula through 1cm incision over skin of the respective site. If necessary, these ports can convert to 5mm by applying adaptor.

Bilateral oophorectomy by endoclip application and electrocautery

In this technique, animals are bilaterally oophorectomised by laparoscopic clip (endoclip) application and electrocautery. Fenestered grasping forceps are placed through right paramedian port and the right ovary is pulled caudally to visualize the right ovarian ligament and vessels properly. The clip applicator preloaded with titanium medium endoclip is inserted through the left paramedian port and the clip is applied around the cranial ovarian ligament including the vessels. A second clip is applied on the uterine horn 0.5 to 1cm away from the ovarian bursa. Laparoscopic scissors are then inserted through the left paramedian port and resection is started from the caudal attachment, cranial to the distal endoclip and close to the ovarian bursa and continued through the uterine horn, broad ligament, and mesovarian attachment. Simultaneous cauterization of the resected site is achieved by applying monopolar or bipolar current through the scissors. To facilitate this procedure, laparoscopic scissors and laparoscopic forceps can be interchanged into their portal placement, whenever require. The total ovarian masses are thus dislodged and removed through one of either 10mm port. The opposite ovary is removed in the same manner.

Ovariohysterectomy by endoclip application and electrocautery

In this technique, animals are subjected to laparoscopic ovariohysterectomy by electrocautery and endoclip application. After achieving sufficient capnoperitoneum and trocar placement in the same manner as described above, fenestrate forceps is inserted through right paramedian port to grasp the right ovary. Clip applicator is inserted through left paramedian port and endoclip is applied around the cranial ovarian ligament and vessels. Simultaneous cauterization and coagulation by applying monopolar/bipolar current and transactions of cranial ovarian ligament is followed by continuous resection of suspensory ligament, ovarian pedicle and broad ligament of uterus up to the level of uterine body. The uterine artery, vein and body, proximal to the cervix are clipped, coagulated and transected. The procedure is repeated in reverse order for left ovary up to the level of cranial suspensory ligament. After completion of procedure the resected genito-uterine portion is taken outside through 10mm port.

Ovariohysterectomy by electrocautery

The technique is same as described above except the endoclip application. By coagulation and cutting of ovario-uterine body at the same level as described above, laparoscopic ovariohysterectomy by electrocautery is done.

Animal is inspected at all resects sites for hemorrhage after the completion of procedure. The telescope is then taken out and the endocamera is detached. Intra abdominal carbon dioxide gas is allowed to escape through the cannula and evacuation is facilitated by both sides abdominal wall compression. The subcutaneous tissue of the umbilical port and skin are apposed with simple interrupted suture in routine manner.

Postoperative Care

The surgical wound/trocar points are regularly dressed in animals using povidone iodine and antiseptic cream until healing. Broad spectrum antibiotic and analgesic should be given to animals for 3-5 days postoperatively. Animal behaviour and all vital parameters should be monitored regularly for at least one week post sterilization.

Complications

The following complications can occur during or after laparoscopic sterilization in bitches.

- Anesthetic complications.
- Air embolism.
- Organ perforation.
- Infection.
- Over distension of capnoperitoneum.
- Cardio-pulmonary arrest.
- Faulty instrumentation.
- Loose endoclipping.
- Faulty cauterization.
- Intraoperative and postoperative bleeding.
- Incomplete removal of utero-ovarian tissue.
- Electrocution during cauterization.

Laparoscopic Sterilization Techniques in Bitch (Bilateral oophorectomy)

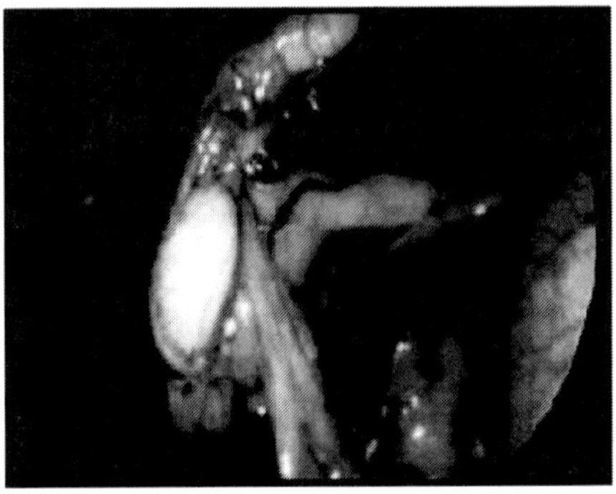

Ovary and mesovarium

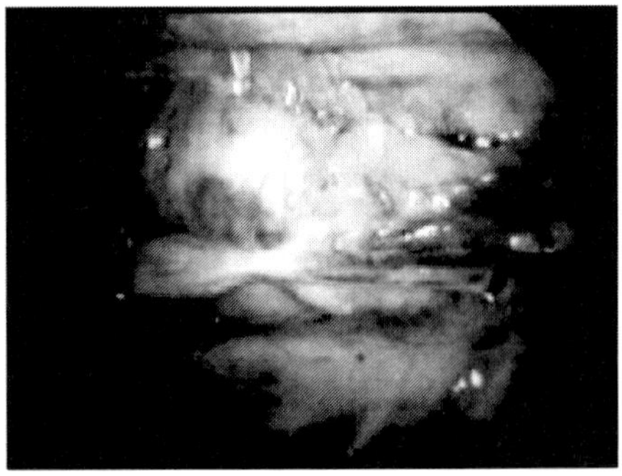

Clip applied both side of the ovary

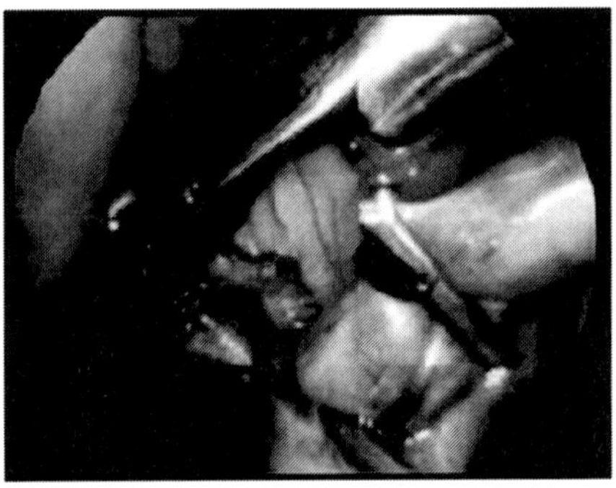

Cauterization and resection of the cranial ovarian attachment

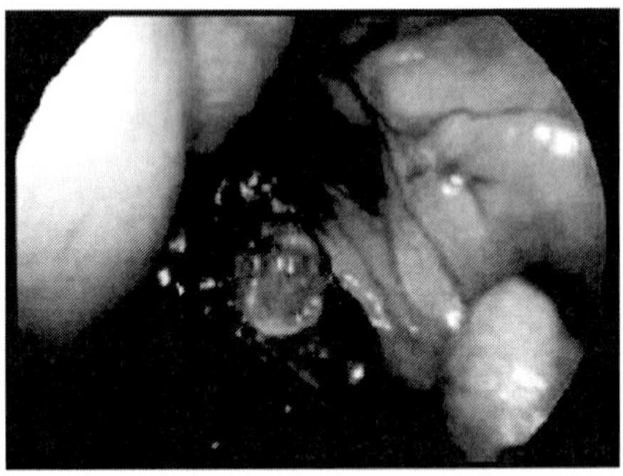

Complete resection of the cranial ovarian attachment

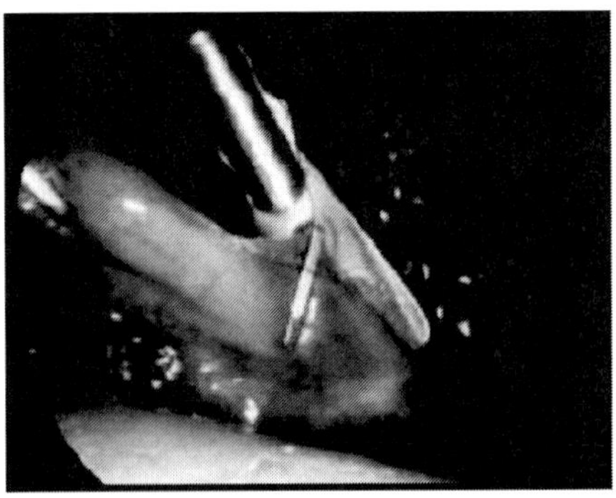

Resection of uterine horn cranial to distal clip

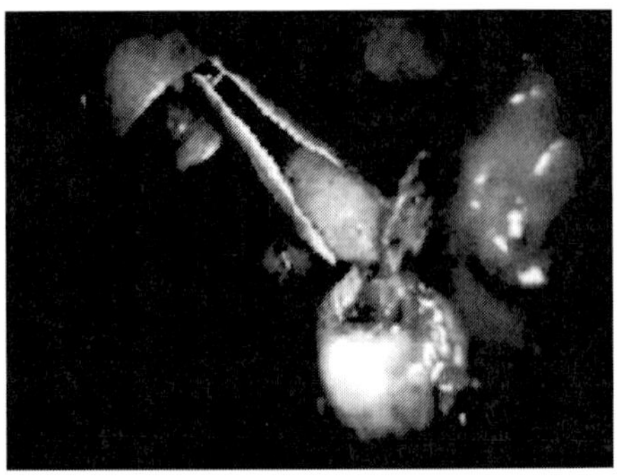

Removal of resected ovary through 10 mm cannula

Laparoscopic Sterilization Techniques in Bitch (Ovariohysterectomy by clip and cautery)

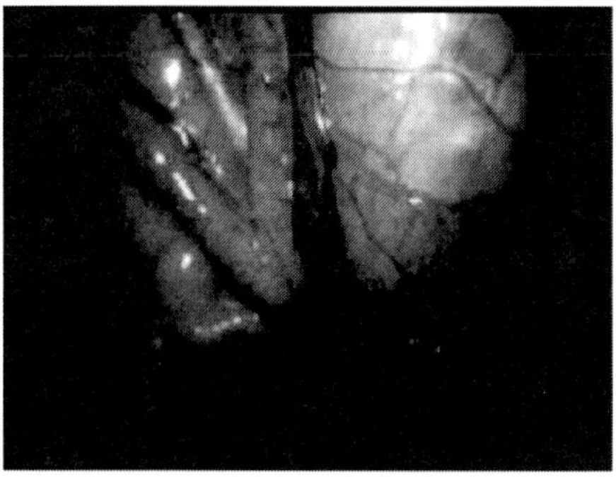

Uterine body and horns

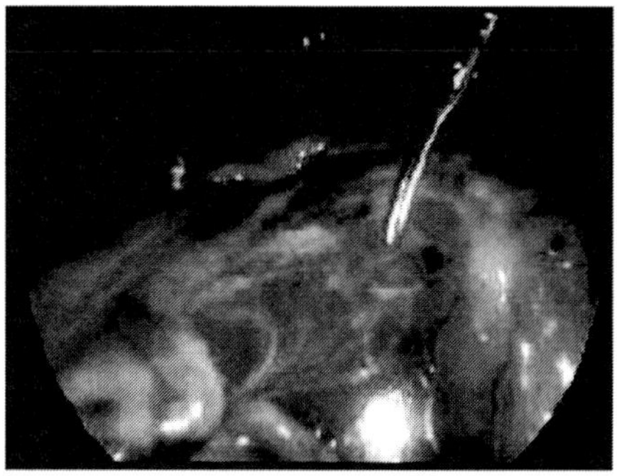

Separation through mesometrium

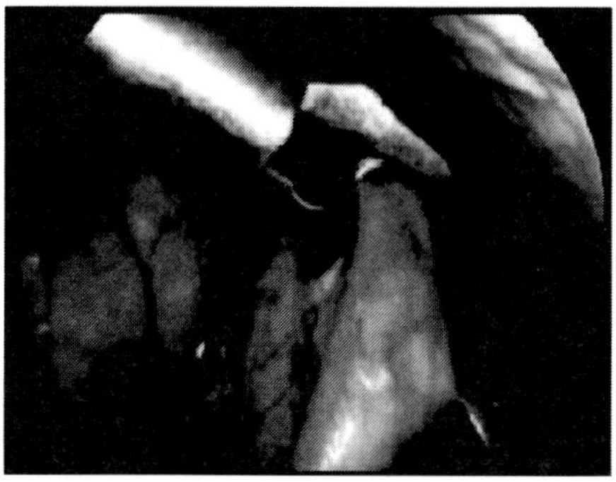

Clipping of uterine body, cranial to cervix

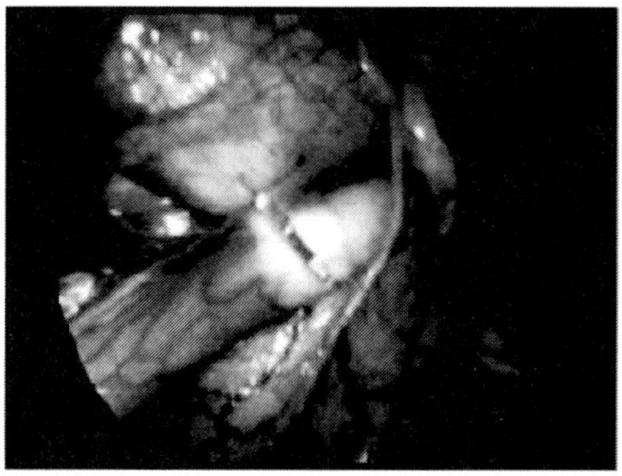

Clipping of uterine body, cranial to cervix

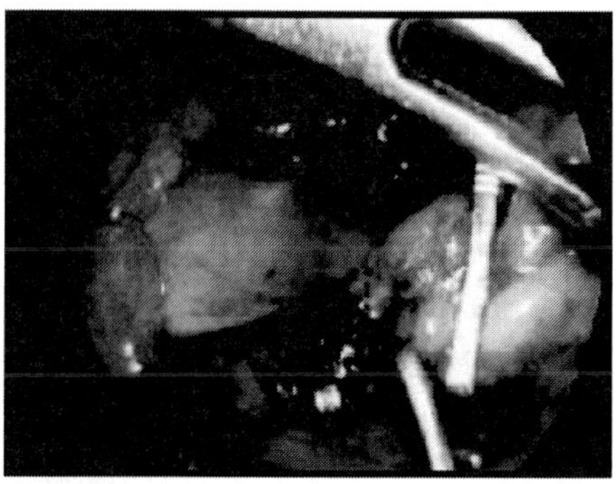

Resection and cauterization of the uterine body after clipping

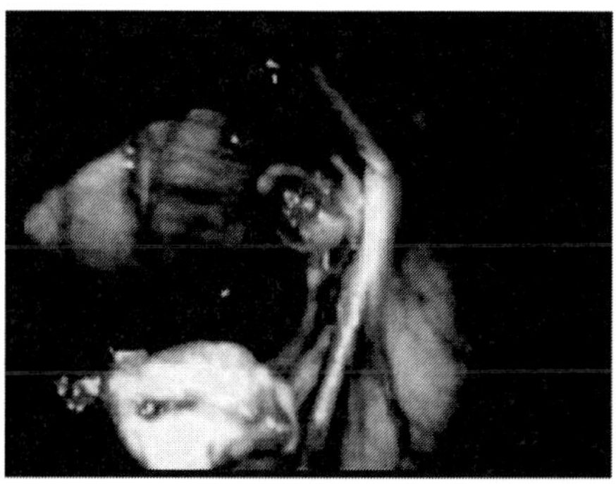

Complete resection of uterine body

Laparoscopic Sterilization Techniques in Bitch (Ovariohysterectomy by electrocautery)

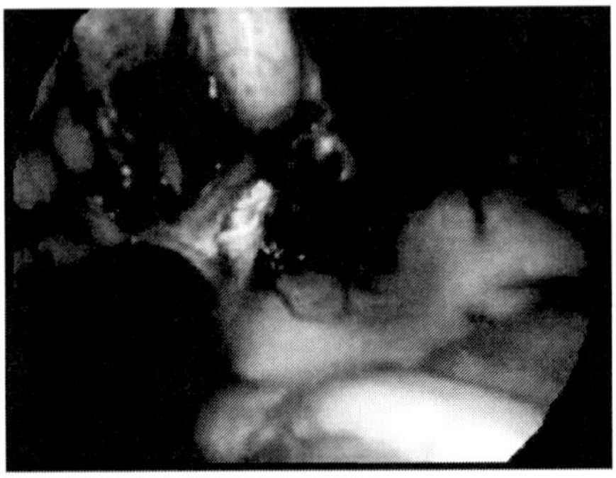

Cauterization and resection of cranial ovarian attachment

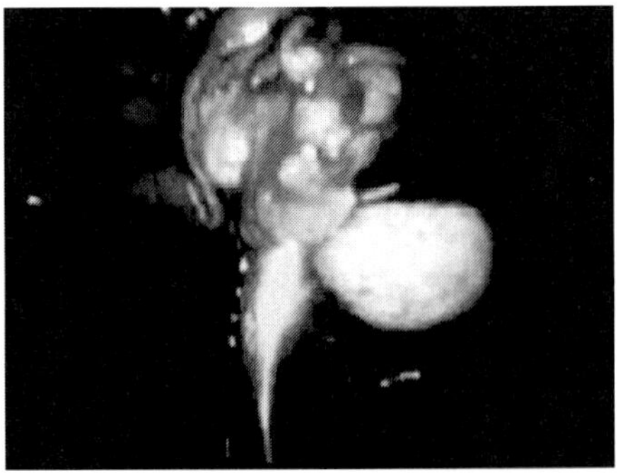

Cauterization and resection of cranial ovarian attachment

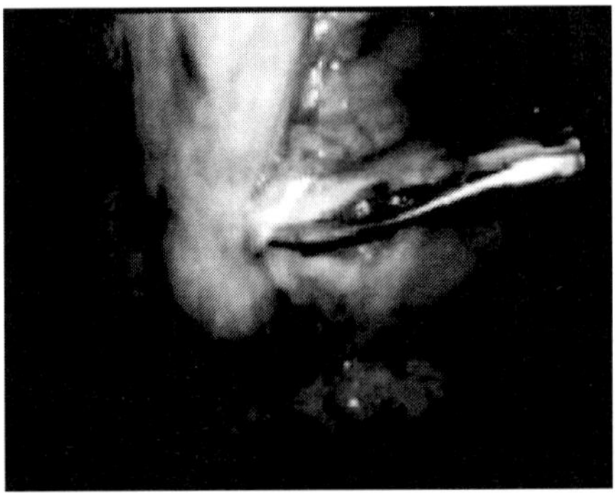

Cauterization and separation of mesometrium

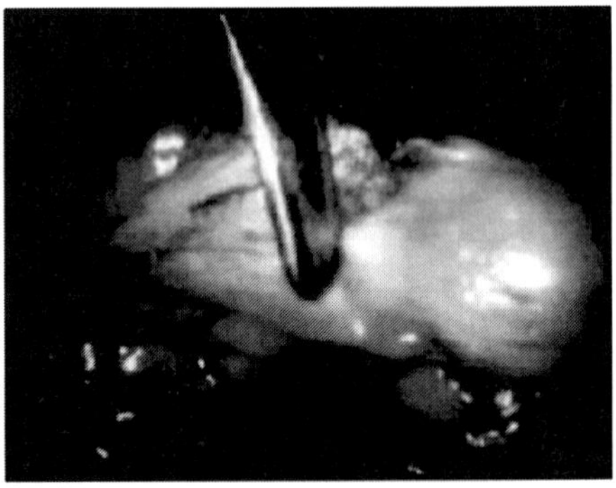

Cauterization and resection of the uterine body

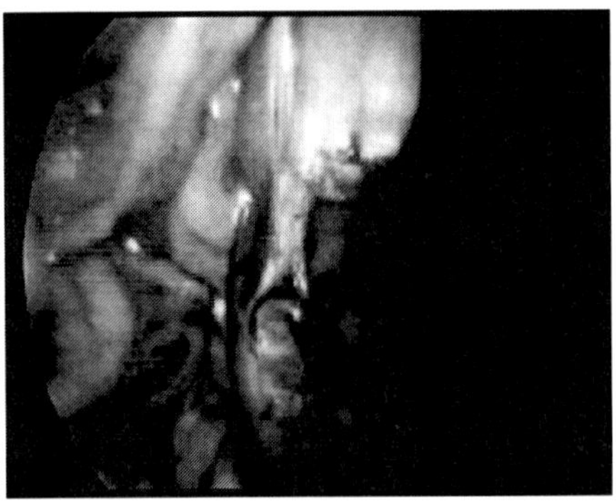

Complete separation of uterine body

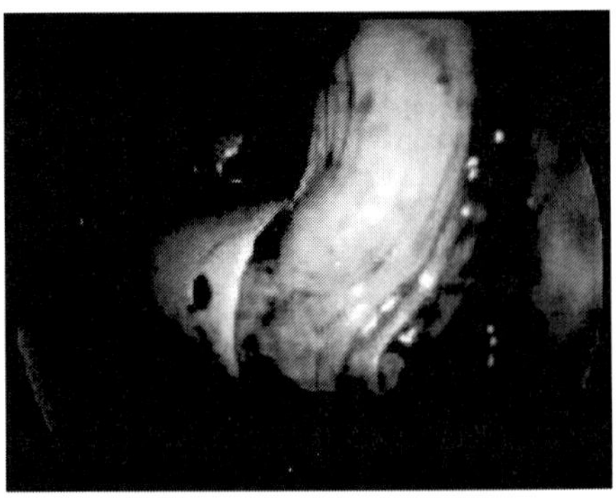

Removal of resected utero- ovarian structure through 10 mm cannula

10

Laparoscopic Sterilization in Male Dogs

Many surgeons have made attempts to develop minimally invasive surgical techniques with minimum blood loss and fewer traumas, to treat the disease process and minimize patient morbidity. Laparoscopic surgery may provide a wide field of its extensive application particularly in surgical sterilization of different animal species. Furthermore, high demographic urban and industrial area requires an effective animal birth control programme, which can overcome the problem of hospitalization, postoperative complications, and the overall cost reduction of operation. The sterilization of (both male and female) is effective measure in controlling the stray dog's problem. Because the sterilization of either male or female alone is not effective and also sterilization of female consume more time when compared to male sterilization. To combat stray dogs in Animal Birth Control (ABC) programme, it is effective to sterilize the male also. Castration of male dogs by conventional open method has many disadvantages and postoperative complications such as hemorrhage, wound dehiscence, infections, maggot infestations and scrotal swellings etc. In a large scale Animal Birth Control programme, the conventional methods of sterilization requires a long period between capture of dogs and their release due to the time taken for the surgical wounds to heal. In this aspect, Keyhole surgery (Laparoscopic surgery) can revolutionize the entire programme, as it needs only very small surgical wound, which usually needs no postoperative care or regular dressings. It also avoids postoperative complications such as wound dehiscence, herniation, etc. and reduces the surgical stress to animal as well as recurring cost of each surgery.

Instrumentation

A. Laparoscopic instruments

- Telescope- 0 or 30^0 forward- oblique, 5 mm telescope.
- Veress needle of 120 mm working length with spring loaded blunt stylet.
- One 5 mm spring loaded safety trocar with two cannula.
- One 10 mm pyramidal tip trocar with two 11 mm cannula.
- One pair fenestered grasping forceps.
- One pair of dissecting and grasping forceps.
- One pair of Metzenbaum curve scissors.
- Two adaptors.
- One 10 mm clip applicator.
- Medium sized titanium endoclips.

B. Laparoscopic equipments

- Electronic, fully automatic CO_2 endoflator with high pressure hose CO_2 gas connector, main cord and silicon tubing set, with CO_2 gas cylinder.
- Xenon or halogen light source having 250 Watt twin lamps of 240 VAC power supply with flexible 5-8 mm fibre optic light cable.
- Digital video camera.
- Medical grade colour monitor.
- Digital video capture system with 3.5 inches floppy disc or compact disc.
- Combined unipolar and bipolar coagulator.

C. General surgical instruments

- A standard general surgical pack containing common surgical instruments.

Surgical Procedure

Laparoscopic surgery is conducted under general anaesthesia. The animal is placed in dorsal recumbency. Fourquarter drapes are placed in mid ventral abdomen from the xyphoid and the pubis. The animals are then placed on a Trendelenburg position to facilitate cranial displacement of the visceral organs.

Vasectomy by cauterization and cutting of vas deferens

A rigid type telescope connected with light source and digital camera is then introduced through cannula. Intraperitoneal organs along with vas deferens are thoroughly visualized. The urinary bladder is identified by its characteristics tortuous structures of blood vessels on it. Then the vas deferens and spermatic artery-vein plexus are visualized. Each vas deferens is observed at the site where both of them joined dorsal to the bladder and they are easily traced to the point where they enter the abdominal cavity at the inguinal ring. The vas deferens is ivory colored and cord like structure. For vasectomy, two ports of 6 mm size are created by using 6 mm trocar-cannula assembly inserted into the peritoneal cavity, under the guidance of telescope, distal to the laparoscopy insertion site and 4-6 cm bilaterally from the ventral midline (distal and lateral to the ventral midline at the inguinal region). Through these ports, the operative instruments are inserted for surgical procedures. The vas deferens is then held by fenestered grasping forceps, inserted through the same side port. The monopolar scissors is inserted through the opposite side port. A monopolar or bipolar current can be used for cutting and cauterization. A piece of 2-3 cm of vas deferens is then resected after coagulation and removed through the cannula. The same procedure is repeated for the opposite vas deferens.

Sterilization by cauterization and cutting of vas deferens plus occlusion of testicular vessels by endoclips

Two 11 mm size ports are created using 10mm pyramidal tip trocar with the 11mm cannula as describe above. The procedure for vas deferens is repeated as mentioned above. After resection and removal of vas deferens, the spermatic artery-vein plexus are identified. Unlike in the scrotum, the vas deferens within the pelvic cavity is not associated with the spermatic artery-vein plexus that courses laterally along the dorsolateral portion of the abdominal wall. The vessels are clipped by applying two titanium clips at a distance of 1-2 cm. The same procedure is repeated for the opposite one. After completing the surgery the telescope and other accessory instruments are removed from the abdominal cavity and intra abdominal gas was allowed to escape through the cannula. One or two simple interrupted sutures are applied to close all the three ports in the abdomen using nylon.

Postoperative care

All the wounds are cleaned and dressed regularly at the portal and incision site with povidone iodine and antiseptic cream. Broad-spectrum antibiotic and analgesic are given for 3-5 days postoperatively.

Complications

- Anesthetic complications.
- Air embolism.
- Over distension of capnoperitoneum.
- Cardio-pulmonary arrest.
- Loose endoclipping.
- Faulty cauterization.
- Intraoperative and postoperative bleeding.

Laparoscopic sterilization techniques in dogs (Vasectomy)

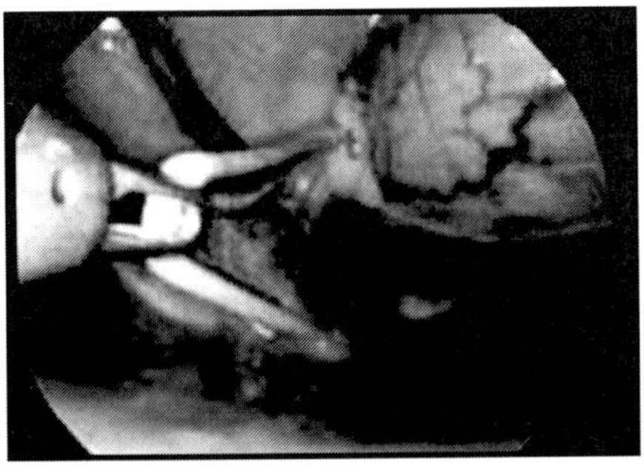

Holding the vas deferens by fenestered grasping forceps for cauterization

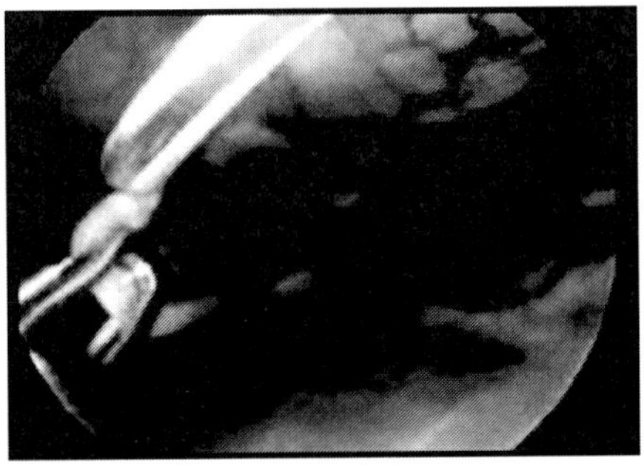

Cauterization of vas deferens by monopolar scissors

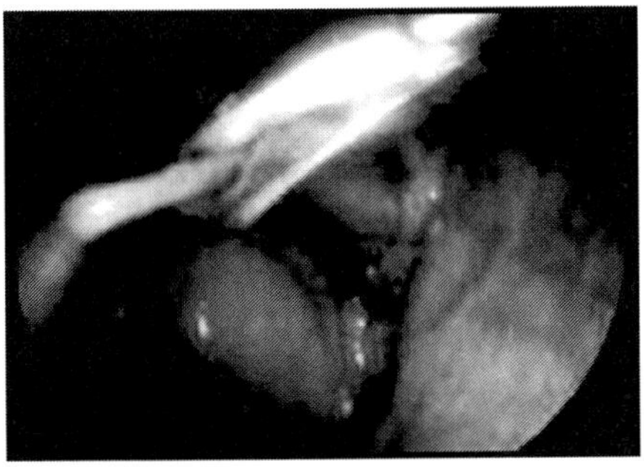

Cutting of vas deferens

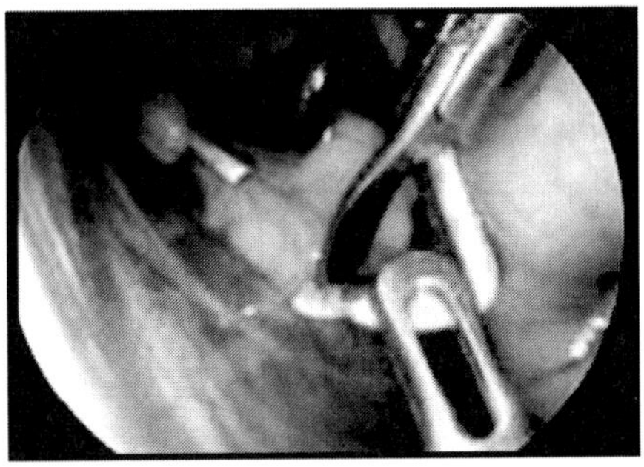

Resection of vas deferens

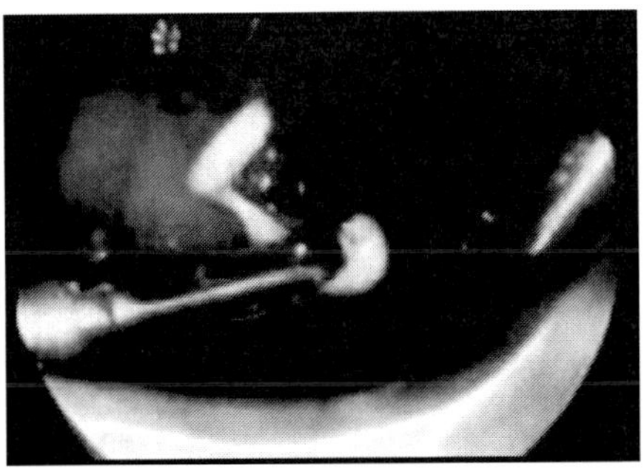

Removal of resected piece of vas-deferens through cannula

Laparoscopic sterilization techniques in dogs (Vasectomy + clipping of spermatic plexus)

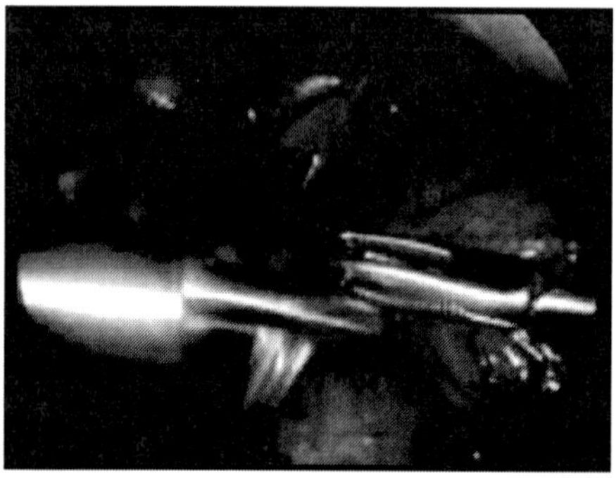

Application of second endoclip in spermatic artery-vein plexus

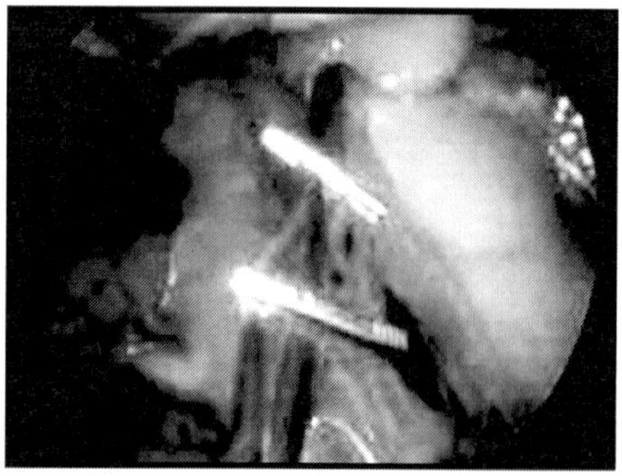

Two endoclips applied to spermatic artery-vein plexus

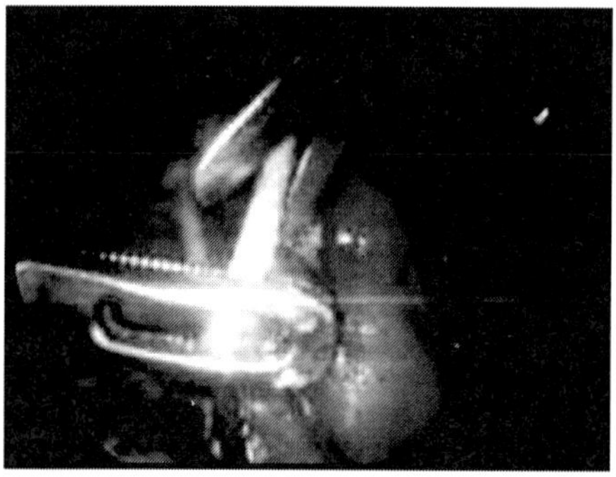

Cauterization and cutting of vas deferens

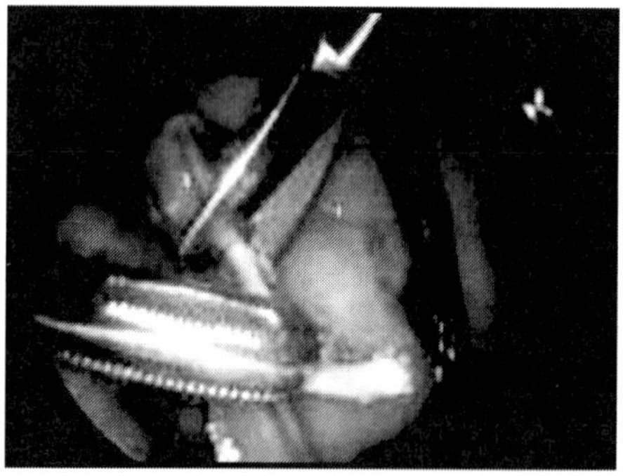

Resection of vas deferens

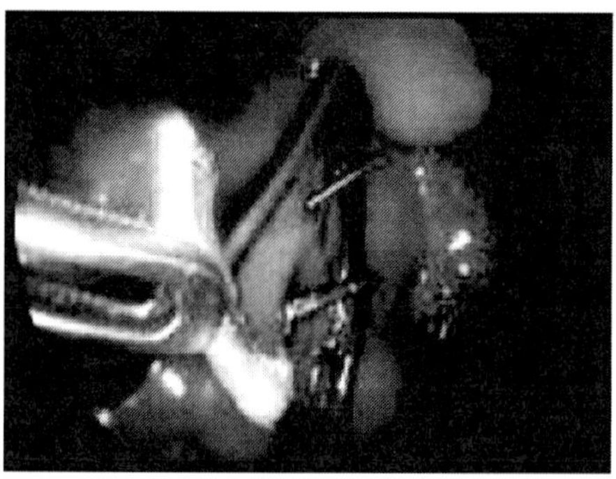

Removal of resected piece of vas deferens outside

11

Laparoscopy in Zoo Animals Practice

Introduction

The most common indication for laparoscopy in zoo animal clinical medicine includes evaluation of liver disorders (e.g. cirrhosis, hepatitis, hepatomegaly), staging for cancer treatment (liver and peritoneal metastases), diagnosis of various peritoneal diseases (e.g. ascites), diagnosis of pelvic soft tissue diseases (e.g. ovarian problem, endometritis, pyometra,) and diseases of spleen and pancreas. The utility of laparoscopy in zoo animal practice is wide and it has been used in almost all the species with encouraging results. Laparoscopy is now most commonly used in zoo animal medicine to examine and biopsy of liver, gall bladder, kidney, spleen, pancreas, ovaries and prostrate. It provides an excellent means for visualizing the surfaces and colour. Even subtle color and texture changes can be readily detected. The liver is generally evaluated through a right lateral mid abdominal approach in canine and feline species of zoo animals. Abnormal gross liver changes that can be readily appreciated include hepatic lipidosis, glycogen leaden liver, metastasis or multifocal neoplasm, nodular hyperplasia, cirrhosis, cholangihepatitis, extra hepatic biliary tract obstruction etc. Using grasping forceps advanced through the second puncture cannula, the biopsy can be obtained quickly and safely in zoo animals. The pancreas can usually be visualized thorough a right abdominal approach and biopsy samples can be safely obtained.

The utility of laparoscopy in zoo animal reproduction is also very wide. Laparoscopy is useful for assessment of ovarian status, ovarian dynamics, ovarian or par ovarian cyst, pregnancy diagnosis, fetal development, uterine pathology, intra uterine treatment, sterilization and for oocyte/embryo collection. Another utility of laparoscopy is sexing of zoo birds. The success of the captive breeding programme at zoological garden always depend on the basic fact of precise identification of sex before pairing. Unlike, few selected procedures laparoscopic sexing forms a vital component in captive breeding programme in case of monomorphic birds among which some birds have been included in the category of endangered species status.

Laparoscopy in exotic birds

Fine diameter rigid endoscopes have been used for diagnostic purposes in exotic birds since the late 1970's. During the decade of the 1980's this technology began to be employed with greater vigor by veterinarians in zoological gardens. The value of minimally invasive surgery that allowed excellent visualization of internal structures even in very small birds becomes popular by zoo veterinarians.

Rigid endoscopes were first employed in birds to visualize the gonads for purpose of sex identification in those species where external characteristics were difficult or impossible to rely upon. The superior resolution and light transmission characteristics of latest model of laparoscope made them superior to other optical systems for avian applications. The unique anatomy of the ovarian respiratory system allowed relatively easy access to many organ systems. Secondary hand instruments can be used to collect biopsies allowing precise targeting of lesions with minimal patient trauma. Lumeig (1987) provided the first comprehensive overviews of endoscopic access points for he bird, using the pigeons as a model.

Anesthesia

Isoflurane gas anaesthesia has become the standard for avian anaesthesia. A number of parenteral agents either singly or in combination, have been used such as ketamine, xylazine, diazepam, midazolam and propofol. However, none of these agents has proven to be as safe or constantly effective as isoflurane for endoscopic procedures. Placing a soft, uncuffed endotraceal tube into the unencumbered glottis readily intubates birds. In most of the exotic species of birds, tracheal rings are complete.

Procedure

The unique anatomy of the avian respiratory system facilitates endoscopic examination. The lungs are fixed to the dorsolateral ribs and do not change significantly in volume during the respiratory cycle. The air sacs of the birds arise from a variety of ostis in the lung and extensively invaginated the coelom. The air sacs provide access to most internal organs without the need for secondary insufflation. The caudal thoracic air sacs are the key entry points to the avian air sac system. The cranial thoracic and abdominal air sacs can be easily accessed from a single entry point into the caudal thoracic sacs via the lateral thoracic wall. This permits inspection of most of the respective right or left hemicoelom. The peritoneum is partitioned by the invagination of the air sacs. The liver is surrounded by the right and left ventral and dorsal hepatic peritoneal cavities. The rest of the abdominal viscera are suspended within the midline intestinal peritoneal cavity as in mammals.

Indications

Ingluvitis	:	Crop burns or trauma.
Abnormal radiographic findings	:	Lung, organomegaly.
Reproductive system	:	Sex determination, infertility.
Respiratory system	:	Pneumoconiosis, pulmonary congestion, granulomatous pleuritis.
Liver	:	Amyloidosis, bile ducts carcinoma, chlamydiosis, liver biopsy.
Heart	:	Pericardial effusion.
Spleen	:	Spleenomegaly, splenic abscess.
Gastrointestinal tract	:	Periventricular dilation.
Kidney	:	Renal disease, shape and size.
Gonads	:	Mature/immature ovary/testicles.

Laparoscopic sexing

The success of the captive breeding programme in an established aviary or at zoological garden depends on the basic fact of precise identification of sex before pairing. Unlike few selected procedures, laparoscopic sexing forms a vital component in captive breeding programme in case of monomorphic birds among which some birds have been included in the category of endangered status, as per wildlife protection act. Laparoscopy sexing technique involves immobilization of avian species and subsequent making one keyhole incision in the selected abdominal area. An appropriate size laparoscope is inserted and gonads are identified accordingly. During sexing by laparoscopy in the mature birds, the ovary is unmistakable as it is covered with maturing follicles, resembles a bunch of grapes and in male birds usually one testis is seen which is smooth in appearance. Immature ovaries are variable in shape and size and difficult to assess in general.

Limitations

- Difficulty in immobilization and restraint of the zoo and wild animals particularly animals in free ranging system.
- Puncture of hollow organs during establishment of pneumoperitoneum.
- Occurrence of gas immobilization after placement of Veres needle within a major vessel, spleen etc.
- Cardiopulmonary compromise due to excessive pneumoperitoneum particularly in small carnivores and artiodactyls species.
- Trocar punctures of visceral organ due to faulty technique.
- Excessive hemorrhage from the biopsy site.
- Disorders of blood coagulation.
- Acute pancreatitis.
- Intestinal obstruction.
- Infection of the abdominal wall.

Conclusions

The laparoscopy techniques adopted in wild and zoo animals are useful in the diagnosis of internal events, intra abdominal surgery, manipulation or treatment of disease and sexing of zoo/wild birds. The most advantageous characteristic of laparoscopy is that it allows direct visualization of abdominal cavity with only minimal (keyhole surgery) and superficial surgical intervention (scar less surgery). Laparoscopy, unlike laparotomy can be performed repeatedly and at frequent intervals in the same zoo/wild animal. However, zoo veterinarians should have clear knowledge of visceral anatomy of different zoo animals and expertization in laparoscopic surgery.

12
Laparoscopy in Animal Physiology

Introduction

Laparoscopy is an operative procedure, performed through a keyhole opening with a rigid telescope that allows visual inspections and biopsy of the peritoneal cavity and its organs. Laparoscopy was first introduced in 1901 in human medicine. It has only been in the last 15 years that laparoscopy has been widely used in various animal species for research, clinical diagnosis and therapeutic purposes. Veterinary laparoscopy was widely used initially in the reproductive physiology in equine, nonhuman primate and various zoo and exotic species. The first clinical application of laparoscopy in dog involved ovarian physiology in the early 1960s, and Lettow reported the first laparoscopic liver biopsy procedure in a dog in 1972. The utility of laparoscopy in animal physiology particularly in reproductive physiology is wide and it has been used in almost all the species with encouraging results.

Instrumentation

The basic equipment for performing laparoscopy in animal physiology includes the different sizes/diameters of laparoscope (telescope) and corresponding trocar-cannula unit, light source, CO_2 gas insufflators, Veress (insufflations) needle and some accessory instruments like scissors, traumatic/atraumatic forceps, biopsy forceps, clip applicator, suction and irrigation pump, fiber optic light cable, unipolar or bipolar coagulator.

Laparoscopy in normal and abnormal physiological evaluation

The laparoscopic procedures are helpful in understanding and evaluating normal and abnormal physiological conditions of different organs.

Liver physiology

A major indication for laparoscopy is to obtain a liver biopsy in animal known or suspected of having liver diseases. The indications are:

- Liver specific biochemistries.
- Liver function test.
- Liver size, texture and colour.
- Hepatic lipidosis, liver has a pale mustard color with friable texture.
- Glycogen laden liver.
- Hepatotoxicit.
- Evaluation of extra hepatic biliary system.
- Metastatic or multifocal neoplasia-raised and discolored tumor nodules with central cavitations or depressions are seen.
- Nodular hyperplasia, multiple raised nodules without central depressions with a yellow fatty appearance.
- Cirrhosis.
- Extra hepatic biliary tract obstruction.
- Liver abscess.
- Liver necrosis.
- Hepatitis.
- Size, volume and position of gall bladder.
- Cytological examination of bile.

- Cholecystocholangiogram (After aspiration of bile from gall bladder, 5-10 ml of iodine contrast agent is directly injected into the gall bladder to visualize the biliary system and to delineate any abnormalities).

Pancreatic physiology

Laparoscopy has been used to evaluate the pancreas in a limited number of cases. The main indications are:

- Pancreatitis.
- Pancreatic tumor.

Spleen physiology

The indications are:

- Normal physiology.
- Spleenomegaly.
- Measurement of splenic pulp pressure (normal 10-15 cm of water).
- Portal hypertension (splenic pulp pressure 20-40 cm of water in chronic liver disease).
- Splenoportography (0.5 ml /kg of iodine contrast directly to the spleen) demonstrate portal blood flow.

Renal physiology

Kidney inspection and biopsy are the major indications for laparoscopic examination of the urinary system.

- Kidney position, shape, size, colour and texture.
- Hydronephrosis.
- Pylonephritis.
- Renal tumors.
- Renal infraction.
- Renal hemorrhag.

- Serosal surface of the urinary bladder.
- Distal portion of the ureters.
- Persistent urachus.
- Ectopic ureter.
- Hydroureter.
- Bladder wall tumor.
- Bladder wall trauma.

Gastrointestinal tract physiology

Laparoscopy has been used to evaluate different organs of gastrointestinal tract particularly in small animals.

- Visualization of stomach.
- Visualization of small and large bowel.
- Visualization of omentum.
- Visualization of intestinal circulation.
- Intestinal intussusceptions/invagination.
- Intestinal torsion.
- Intestinal adhesion.
- Intestinal perforation.
- Intestinal bleeding.
- Intestinal tumor.
- Intestinal foreign body.

Reproductive physiology

The utility of laparoscope in animal reproduction is wide and it has been used in almost all the species with very encouraging results.

- Assessment of ovarian shape, size and colour.
- Assessment of ovarian bursa, pedicle and blood supply.
- Graffian follicle ruptured or non ruptured.

- Assessment of corpus luteum.
- Documentation of ovarian activity.
- *Aspiration of Ovarian or paraovarian cyst*: Ovarian cyst due to hormonal imbalance and not responding to hormonal therapy may be subjected to laparoscopic aspiration. In this procedure a needle of 8-20G is inserted through the abdominal wall. The needlepoint is laparoscopically visualized and guided to the ovarian surface. The needle is inserted into the follicular wall. A syringe is attached to the needle hub and the cystic fluid is completely withdrawn. To prevent the recurrence it is desirable to cauterize the cyst site. Para ovarian cyst can also be treated similarly.
- *Pregnancy diagnosis*: In bitches pregnancy segmental swelling can be seen from 21–25 days of pregnancy. Laparoscopy also helps to determine the litter size by counting the number of sequential bulging in each uterine horn. In bitches, pseudopregnant uterus will have a narrow diameter, light pink coloration and very smooth flaccid appearance.
- *Uterine pathology*: Laparoscopy has been found to be effective for both the detection and confirmation of pathological uterine status. Pyometra, metritis or cystic glandular hyperplasia can be visualized by laparoscopy.
- *Fetal development*: This is facilitated by the use of fetoscope (modified laparoscopy). The instrument has a diameter of 2.7 mm and it is used along with laparoscopy. The procedure involves the insertion of laparoscopy followed by the fetoscopy. The light source of the laparoscopy instrument helps to avoid the vascular and placental areas. The fetoscope can be inserted into the uterine lumen and the fetus can be observed.
- *Sterilization*: Laparoscopy now a day routinely used for sterilizing in dogs and cats. Laparoscopic cutting, stapling or ligation of the oviduct, uterine horn or vas deferens can do sterilization of male and female animals. Laparoscopic oopherectomy is preferred to sterilize and also overcome nuisance associated with estrual behavior.

- *Intrauterine treatment*: Laparoscopy can be used to administer different agents into the uterine lumen. A sterile needle of 16-18 gauge is inserted into the abdominal wall and it is guided laparoscopically towards the point of insertion on the uterine horn. The needle is inserted at 20^0 to 45^0 angles with the plane of the horn. Then small tubing is inserted through the needle. If the tubing resists insertion, the needle likely not in the uterine lumen and should be manipulated until a reasonable length of tubing has been inserted. This arrangement will facilitate uterine flushing, intra uterine administration of semen, drugs etc.
- *Uterine biopsy*: as per intestinal biopsy.
- *Uterine infusion.*
- *Laparoscopic cryptorchidectomy*: Laparoscopy offers excellent visualization of the structures of the inguinal ring and facilitates removal of the abdominally located testis. The internal and external inguinal rings are not invaded, thus the chance of serious complications that may result during open cryptorchidectomy procedures were minimized. Laparoscopic cryptorchidectomy can be performed in dorsal recumbency and standing position.
- *In utero insemination of fresh, chilled or fresh frozen semen*: The technique involves either exteriorization of the uterus as described for the intestinal biopsy or by using a transabdominal technique. For the transabdominal technique involves grasping the uterus with forceps and once stabilized a through-the-needle catheter is placed through the abdominal wall and into the lumen to the uterine body. The needle is removed and semen is then injected through the catheter.

Contraindications

- Peritonitis.
- Diaphragmatic hernia.
- Extensive intra abdominal adhesions.
- Advanced cardiac/pulmonary disease.
- Disorders of blood coagulation.
- Acute pancreatitis.

- Intestinal obstruction.
- Severe portal hypertension.
- Profound ascites.
- Abdominal herniation.

Complications

- Anesthesia related
- Veress needle/trocar insertion
  - Injury to abdominal wall vascular
  - Penetration of organs
  - Perforation of hollow viscus.
- Insufflation
  - Subcutaneous emphysema
  - Peritoneal tenting
  - Inappropriate insufflation
  - Pneumothorax
  - Gas embolism.
- Operative complication
  - Bleedings
  - Tissue injury.
- Technical problems
  - Lack of experience
  - Equipment related problems.

Conclusion

Laparoscopy is a very minimal invasive technique for both diagnostic biopsy and surgical procedures. After the basic technique of laparoscopy is mastered and the appropriate indication learned these procedures become an easy and rewarding addition to any small animal surgery in veterinary practice.

References

Ajith, P., Maiti, S.K., Kumar, N. and Sharma, A.K. (2010) Comparative evaluation of laparoscopic vs. ultrasound guided liver biopsy techniques in canines, Indian Journal of Animal Sciences, 80:405-409.

Altobelli LC et al., (1980) LaprocatorTM Preventive Care and Maintenance. JHPIEGO Corporation: Baltimore, MD.

Anburaja, M., Kumar, N., Maiti, S.K., Sharma, A.K., Dimri, U. and Kataria, M. (2009) Laparoscopic sterilization Vs open method sterilization in dogs: A comparison of two techniques, Turkish Journal of Veterinary and Animal Sciences, 33:427-436.

Anderson (1937) Cited by Magne, M.L. (1990) Laparoscopy: Instrumentation and Technique. In: Small Animal Endoscopy (Tams, T.R. editor) C.V. Mosby Company. St. Louis, pp. 367-375.

Bozzini, Philip (1804) Cited by Magne, M.L. (1990) Laparoscopy: Instrumentation and Technique. In: Small Animal Endoscopy (Tams, T.R. editor) C.V. Mosby Company. St. Louis, pp. 367-375.

Bunch, S.E., Polak, D.M. and Hornbuckle, W.E. (1985) A modified laparoscopic approach for liver biopsy in dogs. J. Am. Vet. Med. Asso. 187: 1032-1035.

Choudhuri, S., Dutta, A., Varshney, J.P. and Maiti, S.K. (2006) Clinico-electro-graphic and laparoscopic evaluation of a distended abdomen of a Labrador, 25th Annual conference of ISVM, Bangalore, Abstract no-P-5. P-137.

Dharmaceelan, S., Ganesh, T.N. and David, W.P. (2000) Laparoscopic sterilization in bitches; comparison of three techniques. Indian J. Vet. Surg. 21: 65-68.

Dutta, A., Maiti, S.K., Ajith, P. and Kumar, N (2010) Evaluation of different laparoscopic sterilization techniques in a canine birth control program. Turkish Journal of Veterinary and Animal Sciences 34: 393-402.

Ganesh, T.N. (2001) Techniques of laparoscopy for examination of visceral organs in cattle. 5th National Training Course on Laparoscopy in Veterinary Practice, Departments of Clinics, Madras Veterinary College, Tamil Nadu Veterinary and Animal Sciences University, Chennai.

Ganesh, T.N. and Dharmaculan, S. (1998) Laparoscopic ovariectomy in dogs. XXII Annual Congress of ISVS (Bhubaneswar).

Ganesh, T.N., Dharmacuhan, S., Rameshkumar, B., Suresh, R.V., Vasu, K. and Pattabiraman, S.R. (1997) Laparoscopy and guided biopsy of hepatoma affected liver in dog. In Souvenir of XXI Annual Congress of ISVS (Palampur).

Ganesh, T.N., Joseph, C., Veerapandian, C., Vasu, K., Thilagar, S. and Archibald, W.P.D. (2001) Laparoscopic diagnosis of certain diseases in dogs. XXV Annual Congress of ISVS (Hissar).

Ganesh, T.N., Nagarajan, B., Rameshkumar, B. and Danapalan, S. (1998) Laparoscopy and guided biopsy of liver affected with cirrhosis in a dog. XXII Annual Congress of ISVS (Bhubaneswar).

Ganesh, T.N., Saravanan, D., Balasubramanian, S., Sridhar, R. and Pattabiraman, S.R. (1999) Laparoscopic observation of tuberculous lessions in a cow. XXIII Annual Congress of ISVS (Chennai).

Geetze (1926) Laparoscopy : Instrumentation and Technique. In: Small Animal Endoscopy (Tams, T.R. editor) C.V. Mosby Company. St. Louis, pp. 367-375.

Grauer, G.F., Twedt, D.C. and Mero, K.N. (1983) Evaluation of laparoscopy for obtaining renal biopsy specimens from dogs and cats. J. Am. Vet. Med. Assoc. 183: 677-679.

Harrison, G.J. (1978) Endoscopic examination of avian gonadal tissue, Vet Med Small Anim Clin, 73: 479-484.

Harrison, R.M. and Wildt, D.E. (1980) Animal Laparoscopy, Williams and Williams, Baltimore, USA.

Ingram, K.A. (1980) Otoscopic technique for sexing birds. In, Current Veterinary Therapy, VII, Philadelphia. W.B. Saunders Co.

Johnson, G.F. and Twedt, D.C. (1977) Endoscopy and laparoscopy in the diagnosis and management of neoplasia in small animals. Vet Clin North America, 7: 77-92.

Jones D.M. et al., (1984) Sex determination of monomorphic birds by fiber optic Endoscopy, Vet Rec., 115: 596-598.

Joseph, C. (2001) Techniques for laparoscopic examination of visceral organs in dogs. 5th National Training Course on Laparoscopy in Veterinary Practice, Departments of Clinics, Madras Veterinary College, Tamil Nadu Veterinary and Animal Sciences University, Chennai.

Karsai, F. (1994) Diagnosis and treatment of hepatic diseases of dogs. Magyar Allatorvosok Lapja, 49: 453-459.

Kelling (1904) Laparoscopy : Instrumentation and Technique. In: Small Animal Endoscopy (Tams, T.R. editor) C.V. Mosby Company. St. Louis, pp. 367-375.

Kumar, N., Amburaja, M., Sharma Ashok. K., Maiti, S.K., Dimri, U. and Kataria, M. (2006) Intra-abdominal laparoscopic vasectomy in male dogs: a new technique. 30th Annual Conference of ISVS, Bidar, Abstract no-4: 8, P-23.

Kumar, N., Dubey, A. K., Singh, G. R., Maiti, S.K. and Sharma, A.K. (2006) Laparoscopic assisted tube cystectomy in clinical cases of complete urinary obstruction in goats. 93rd Indian Science Congress, Hyderabad, Section-Veterinary Sciences, Abstract no-95.

Lettow, E. (1972) Laparoscopic examinations in liver diseases in dogs. Vet. Med. Rev. 2: 159.

Magne, M.L. (1999) Laparoscopy: Instrumentation and Technique. In: Small Animal Endoscopy (Tams, T.R. editor) C.V. Mosby Company. St. Louis, pp. 397-408.

Maiti, S.K. (2002) Management of different surgical conditions in wild and zoo animals. In, Healthcare and Management of Zoo Animals, Published by Society for Conservation of Flora and Fauna, pp-28-43.

Maiti, S.K. (2002) Useful information on wild animals. In, Healthcare and Management of Zoo Animals, Published by Society for Conservation of Flora and Fauna, pp-109-111.

Maiti, S.K. (2004) Prospect of laparoscopic surgery in zoo animal practice, Indian Wildlife Year Book, Vol-3, pp-75-78.

Maiti, S.K. (2009) Minimal invasive surgery in canines. Paper presented at 2nd Federation of Asian Small Animal Veterinary Association (FASAVA) World Congress, Bangkok, Thailand, Congress Proceedings, p-522.

Maiti, S.K. (2009) Laparoscopic diagnosis of some critical clinical cases. Paper presented at 2nd Federation of Asian Small Animal Veterinary Association

(FASAVA) World Congress, Bangkok, Thailand, Congress Proceedings, p-522.

Maiti, S.K. (2010) Laparoscopic-assisted diagnosis and surgical management of different intraperitoneal disorders in dogs. Paper presented at 35th World Small Animal Veterinary Association (WSAVA) World Congress, Geneva, Switzerland, Congress Proceedings, BOP-3, p-84.

Maiti, S.K., Ajith, P. Dutta, A. and Kumar, N. (2013) Laparoscopic and histopathological diagnosis of different intra-abdominal lesions in dogs, Indian Journal of Animal Sciences 83: 488-490.

Maiti, S.K., Ajith, P., Dutta, A, Kumar, N., Sharma, A.K. and Sharma, A (2008) Laparoscopic liver biopsy through cauterization in dogs. The Indian Journal of Animal Sciences 78: 1338-1341.

Maiti, S.K., Ajith, P., Dutta, A., Kumar, N., and Sharma, A.K (2011) Laparoscopic-assisted cholecystocentesis and cholecystocholangiography in canines. Journal of Applied Animal Research 39: 29-32.

Maiti, S.K., and Dutta, A. (2008) Evaluation of different sterilization techniques in canine birth control programme. Paper presented at 33rd World Small Animal Veterinary Association (WSAVA) World Congress, Dublin, Ireland, Congress Proceedings, p-694.

Maiti, S.K., Dutta, A, Khimta, S., Bhadane, B. and Kumar, N. (2009) Laparoscopic diagnosis of splenic tumour in a dog and its surgical management. Paper presented at 33rd Annual Conference of Indian Association for Veterinary Surgery, Ludhiana, Conference Proceedings, SAP-1, p-75.

Maiti, S.K., Dutta, A., Ajith, P., Kumar, N., Sharma, A. K. and Sharma, Ashok. K. (2006) The use of laparoscopy as a diagnostic tool in canine intraperitoneal disorders. 30th Annual Conference of ISVS, Bidar, Abstract no-4: 7, P-22.

Maiti, S.K., Dutta, A., Ajith, P., Kumar, N., Sharma, A.K. and Singh, G.R (2008) Laparoscopy for direct examination of internal organs in small animals. Journal of Applied Animal Research 33: 201-204.

Maiti, S.K., Dutta, A., Tiwary, R., Ajith, P., Kumar, N. and Singh, G.R. (2005) Laparoscopic diagnosis of intra-abdominal pathologies in canines. 29th Annual Conference of ISVS, IVRI, Abstract no-4: 25, P-47.

Maiti, S.K., Dutta, A., Varshney, J. and Kumar, N. (2013) Effect of carbon dioxide pressure gradients in capnoperitoneum for laparoscopic examination in dogs. World Journal of Laparoscopic Surgery 6: 53-62.

Maiti, S.K., Kumar, N., Dutta, A., Ajith, P., Sharma, A.K. and Sharma, Ashok, K (2007) The use of laparoscope for the diagnosis of intraperitoneal disorders and sterilization in dogs. Paper presented at 32nd World Small Animal Veterinary Association (WSAVA) World Congress, Sydney, Australia, Congress Proceedings, p-369.

Maiti, S.K., Kumar, N., Khimta, S., Bhadane, B., Sharma, A.K., Sharma, Anil, K (2007) Laparoscopic diagnosis of hepatic liposarcoma and spelinic haemangiosarcoma in dogs. Paper presented at 31st Annual Conference of Indian Association for Veterinary Surgery, Jammu, Conference Proceedings, 8:20, p-104.

Maiti, S.K., Kumar, N., Sharma, A.K. (2009) Laparoscopic diagnosis and surgical management of intestinal intussusceptions in a dog. The Indian Veterinary Journal 86: 953-954.

Maiti, S.K., Parti, M.K., Singh, M., N. Kumar and Singh, G.R., (2004) Laparoscopic diagnosis of intestinal intussusception and its surgical management in a dog. 28th Annual Congress of ISVS, Jabalpur.

Maiti, S.K., Singh, G.R., Kumar, N., Sharma, A.K. and Hoque, M. (2004) Laparoscopy liver biopsy through cauterization in small animals, 28th Annual Congress of ISVS, Jabalpur.

Maiti, S. K. (2007) "Studies on Laparoscope Guided Biopsy in Animals". Final Report of Indian Council of Agricultural Research, New Delhi, ad-hoc project submitted as Principal Investigator (PI).

McDonald, S.E. (1982) Special sexing of birds by laparoscopy. Calcif. Vet., 5: 16-22.

Megala (1967) Laparoscopy : Instrumentation and Technique. In: Small Animal Endoscopy (Tams, T.R. editor) C.V. Mosby Company. St. Louis, pp. 367-375.

Murray, M.J., Schildger, B. and Taylor, M. (1998) Endoscopy in birds, reptiles, amphibians and fish. Endo-press, Germany, pp 7-28.

Rawlings, C.A (2002) Laparoscopic-assisted gastropexy. J Am Anim Hosp Assoc, 38: 15-19.

Rothuizen, J. (1985) Laparoscopy in small animal medicine. Vet Quarterly, 3: 225-228.

Richter, K.P. (2001) Laparoscopy in dogs and cats. Vet Clin North Am Small Anim Pract, 4: 707-727.

Tams, T.R. (1990) Small Animal Endoscopy, C.V. Mosby Co, St Lewis, USA.

Taylor, M. (1993) Diagnostic application of a new endoscopic system for birds. Proc. Eur. Conf. Avian. Med Surg, Utrecht, NL, pp-127-131.

Thilagar, S., Ganesh, T.N., Joseph, C. and Kumaresan, A (2001) Manual of 5th National training course on laparoscopy in veterinary practices. Madras Veterinary College, Chennai.

Twedt, D.C., and Johnson, G.F. (1977) Laparoscopy in the evaluation of liver disease in small animals. American J Dig. Dis. 22: 571-580.

Twedt, D.C (1999) Laparoscopy of the liver and pancreas. In: Tams, T.R., Editor, Small Animal Endoscopy. 2nd ed, Missouri: C.V. Mosby Co. p 44-60.

Twedt, D.C (2009) Laparoscopy. Lecture in Pre-Congress Seminar, 2nd Federation of Asian Small Animal Veterinary Association (FASAVA) Congress; 2009, November, Bangkok, Thailand.

Veerapandian, C. (2001) Application of laparoscopy in animal reproduction and embryo transfer technology. 5th National Training Course on Laparoscopy in Veterinary Practice, Department of Clinics, Madras Veterinary College, Tamil Nadu Veterinary and Animal Sciences University, Chennai.

Wackes, J. (1996) Laparoscopic and thoracoscopic biopsies in the dog and cat. Kleintierpraxis 41: 411-418.

Wakankar, C.C., Kulkarni, V. and Chariar, V.M. (1999) Laparoscopic ovario-hysterectomy in eight bitches, XXIII Annual Congress of ISVS (Chennai).

Wildt, D.E., Kinney, G.M. and Seager, S.W.J. (1977) Laparoscopy for direct observation of internal organs of the domestic cat and dog. Am. J. Vet. Res. 38: 1429-1432.

Wolf R. (1984) Instruction Manual: Gynecological Laparoscopy Instruments. (Ref. E1-05-82). Richard Wolf Medical Instruments Corp.:Rosemont, IL.

❑❑❑

Colour Plates

Chapter 3: Instrumentation

Instrumentation and procedures

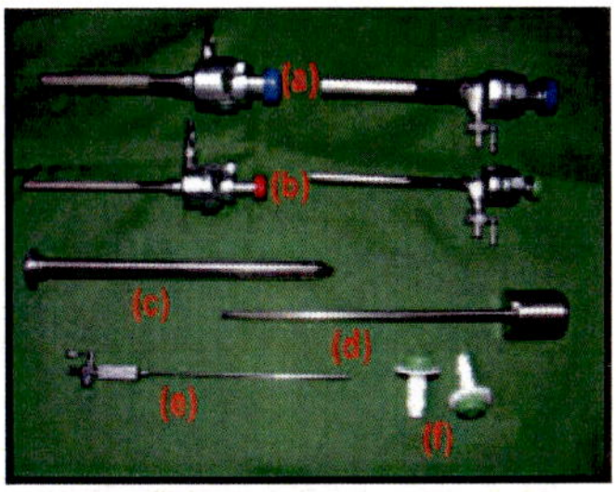

Instruments for laparoscopy (a) 10 mm cannula (b) 5 mm cannula (c) 10 mm pyramidal tip trocar, (d) 5 mm safety trocar, (e) Veress needle (f) Adapter

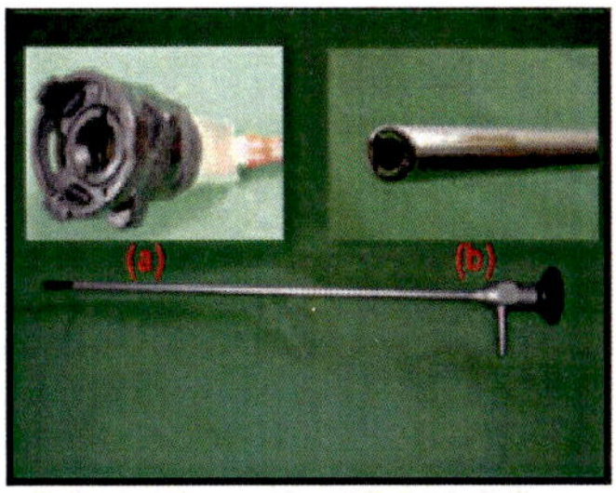

5 mm 30 forward-oblique telescope (a) Endocamera (b) Telescope tip

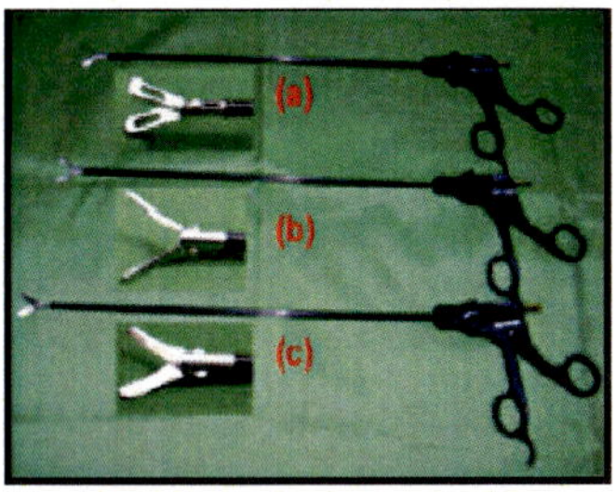

Laparoscopic instruments
(a) Fenestered grasping forceps,
(b) Traumatic forceps,
(c) Monopolar scissors

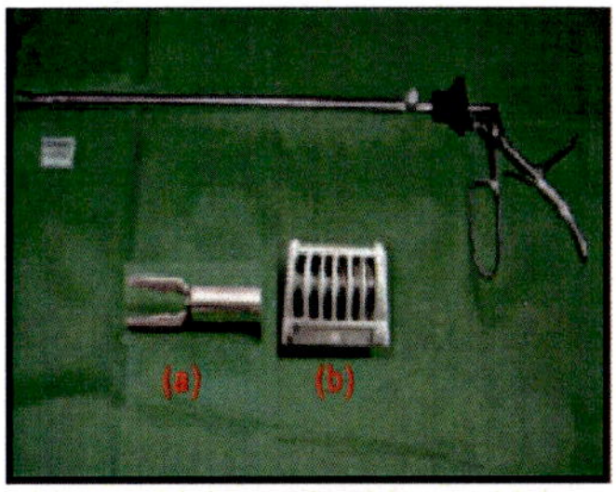

Endoclip applicator (a) Tip of clip applicator (b) Titanium clip cartridge

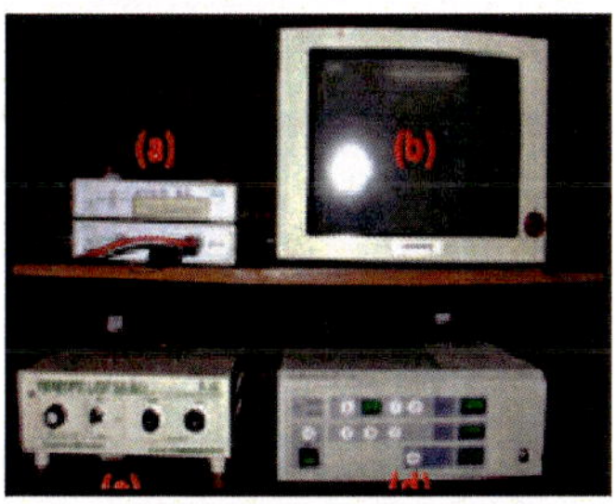

Laparoscopic equipment's
(a) L-cap, (b) Television monitor
(c) Halogen light source,
(d) Endoflator

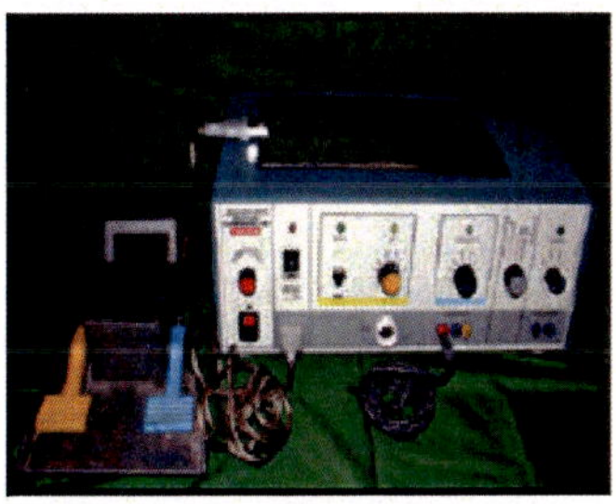

Electrocautery unit

Instrumentation and procedures

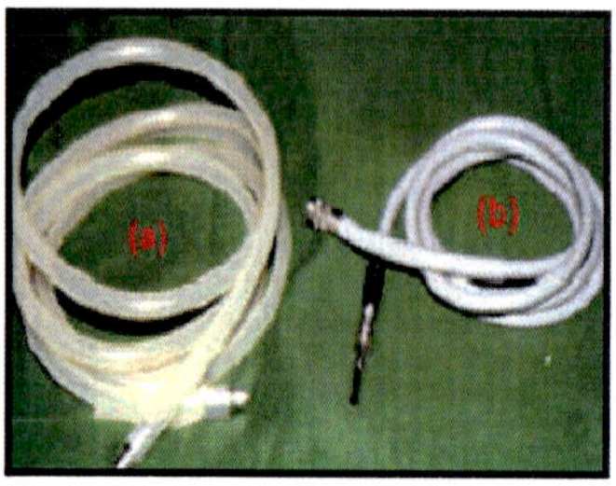

Laparoscopy equipment's (a) CO_2 gas hose, (b) Fibre optic cable

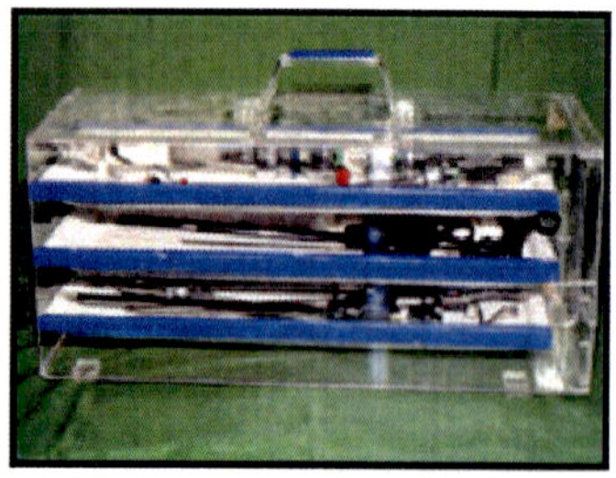

Closed formalin chamber

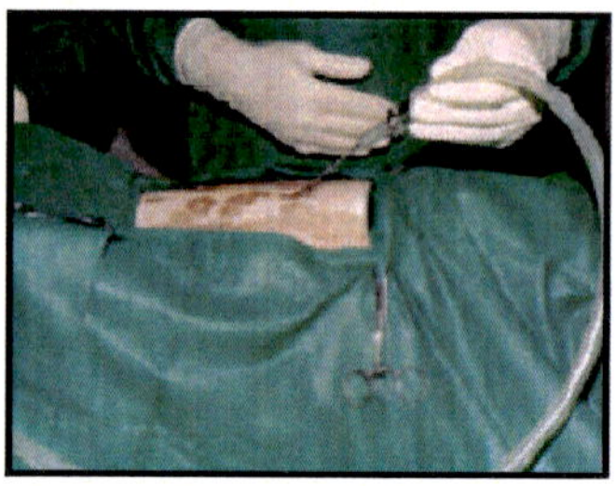

Insertion of Veress needle

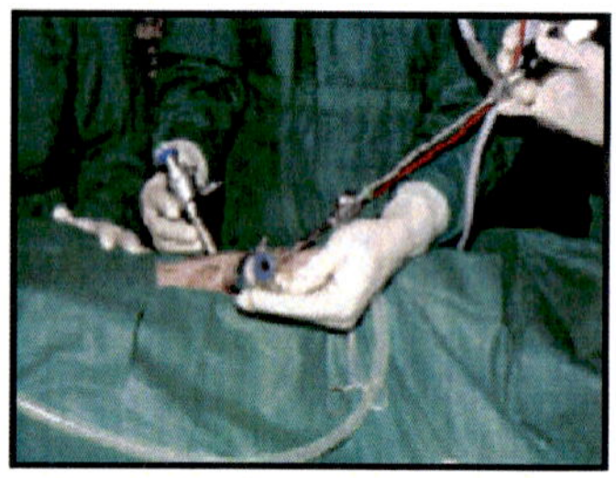

Outside arrangement of three trocars

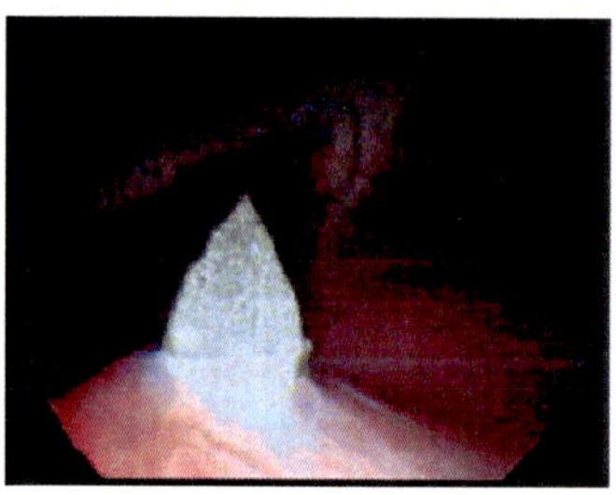

Entry of trocars under laparoscopic guidance

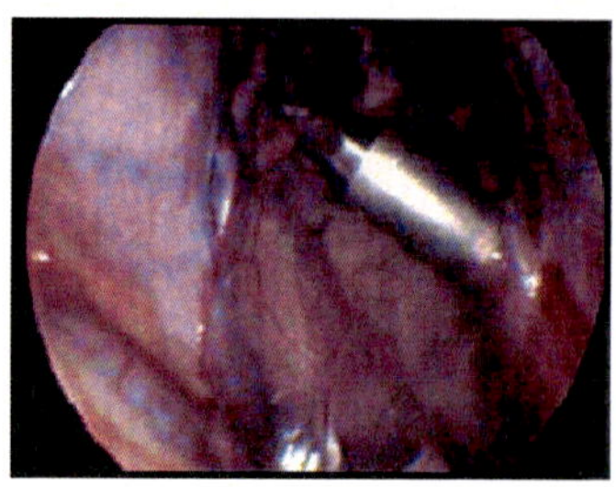

Entry of trocars under laparoscopic guidance

Chapter 6: Techniques for Laparoscopic Examination

Laparoscopic view of different peritoneal organs in goat

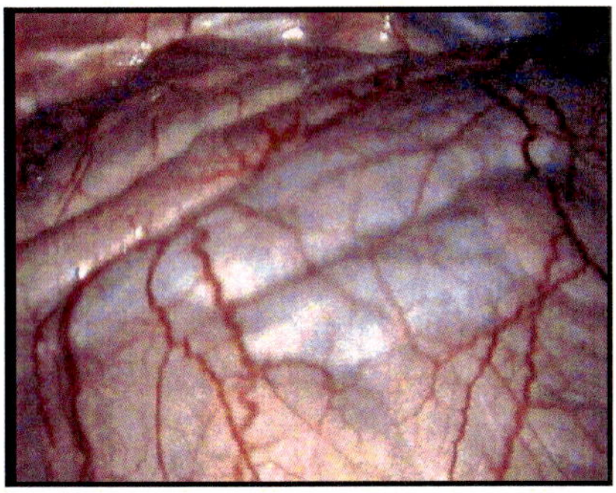

Small Intestine

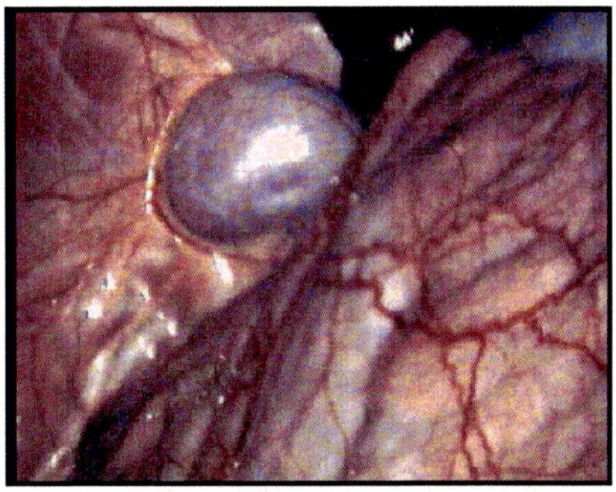

Kidney

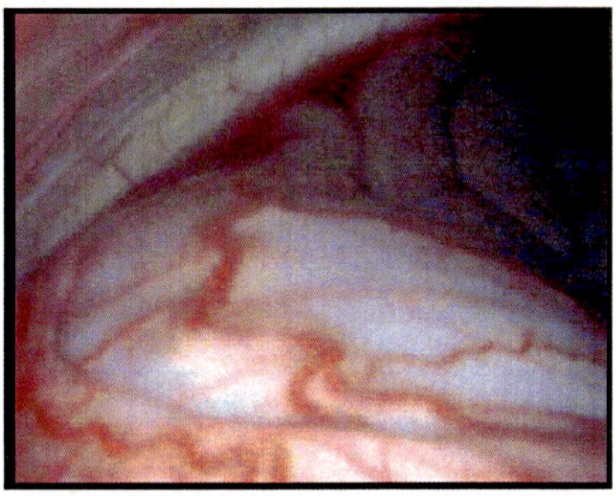

Urinary Bladder

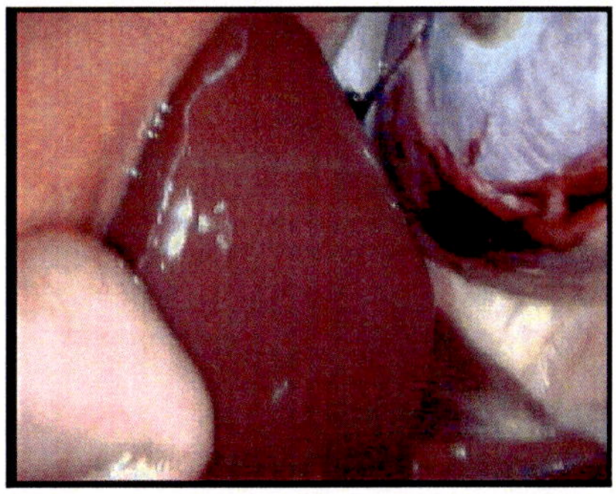

Liver

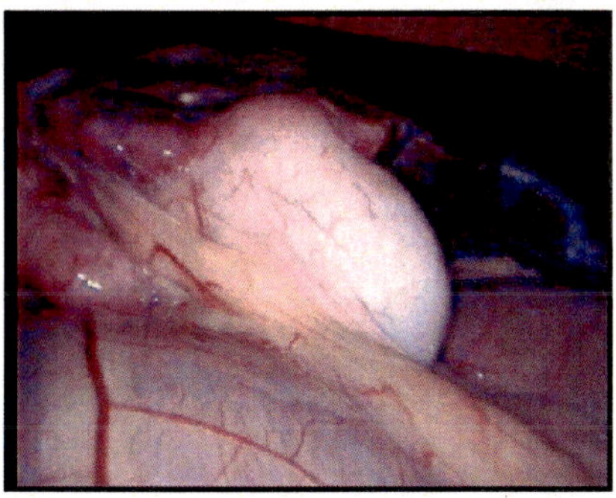

Gall Bladder

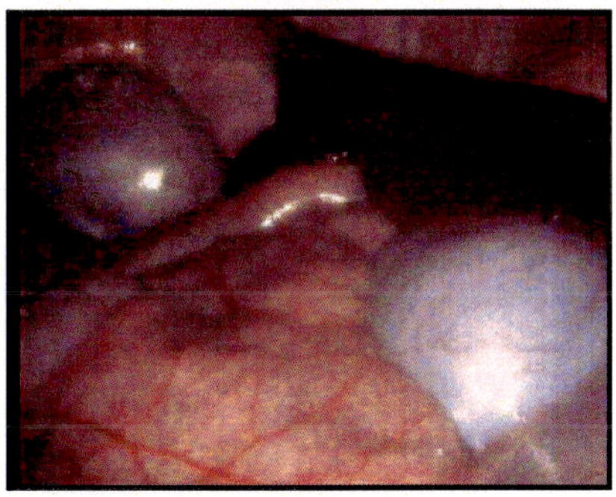

Abomasum

Laparoscopic view of different peritoneal organs in rabbit

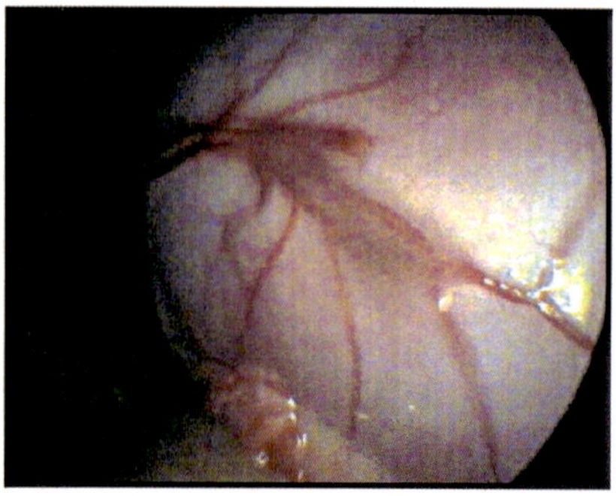

Stomach

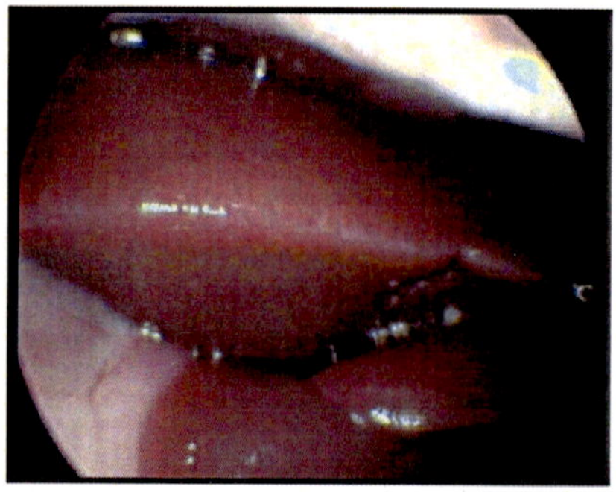

Liver

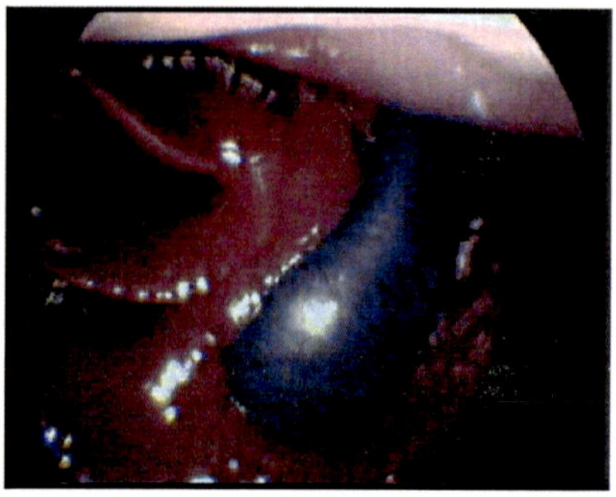

Gall Bladder

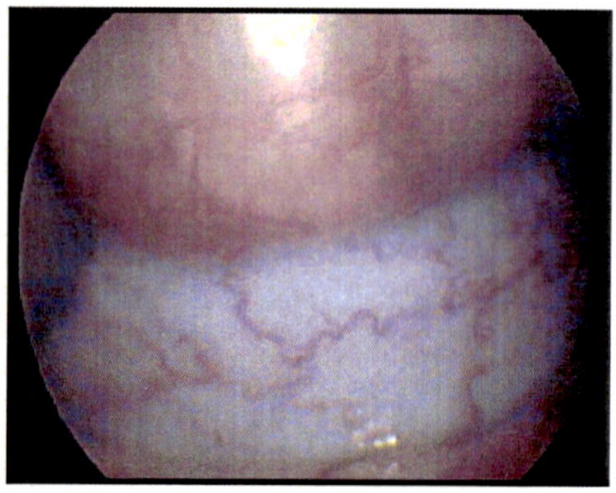

Urinary Bladder

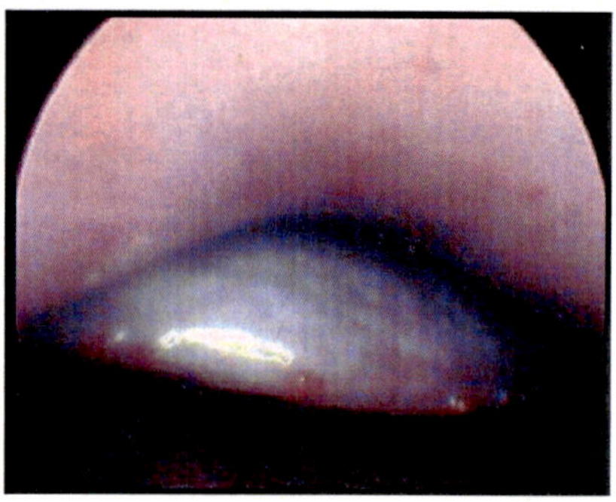

Spleen

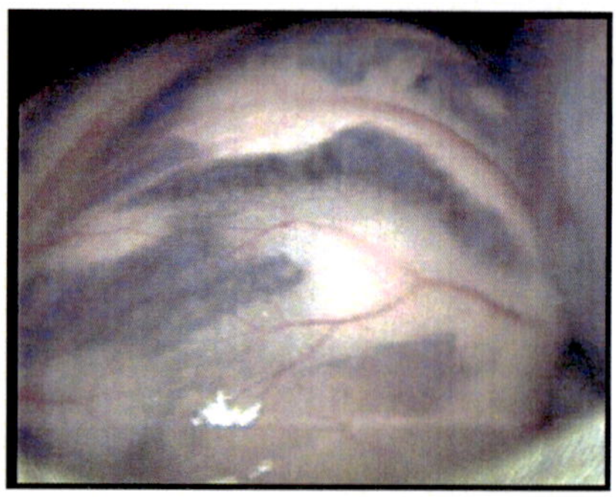

Large Intestine

Laparoscopic visualization of different organs in dog

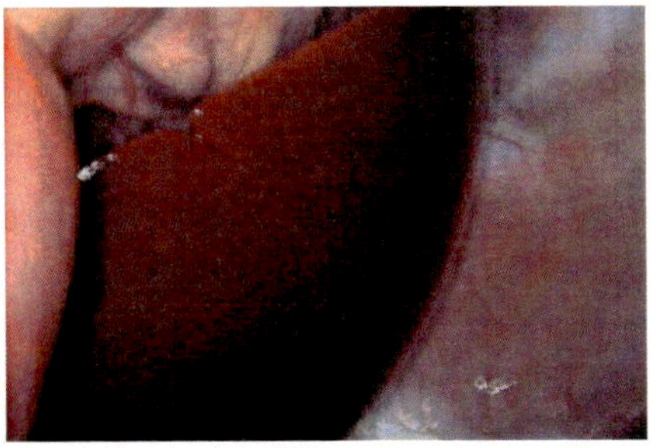

Liver

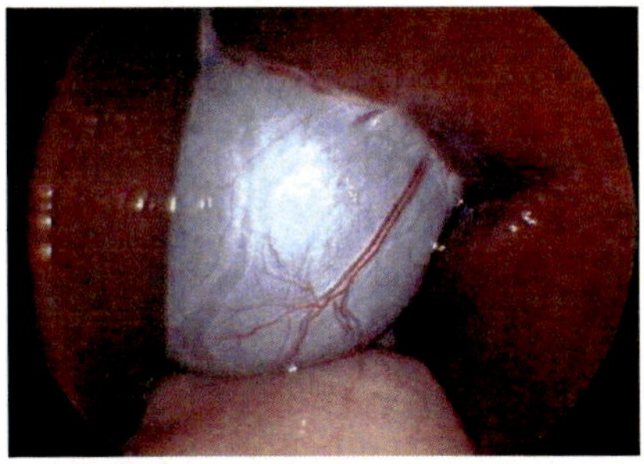

Gall Bladder

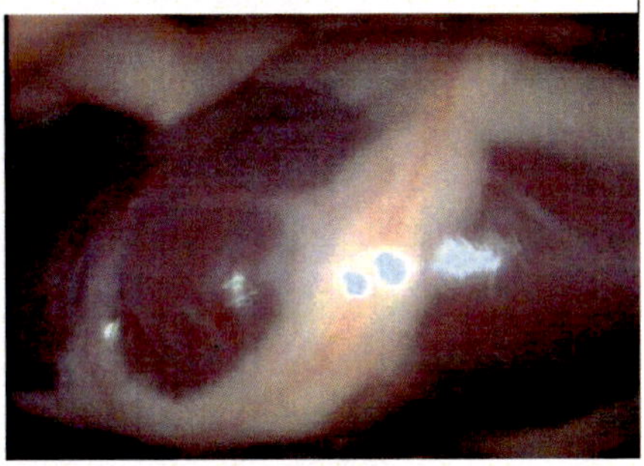

Kidney

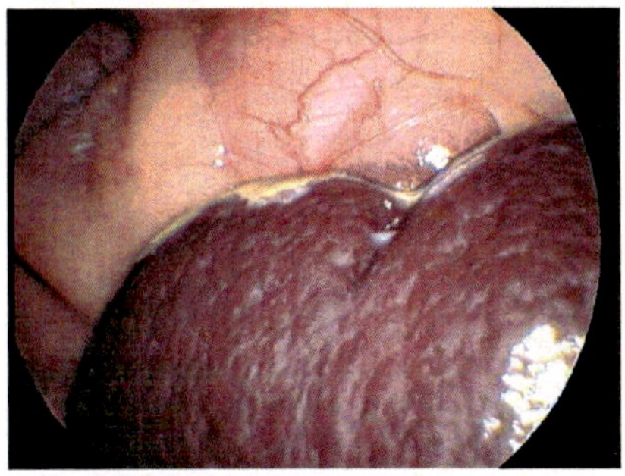

Spleen

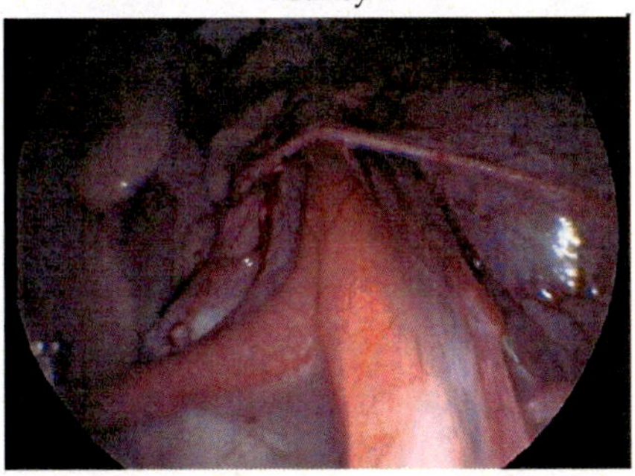

Uterus

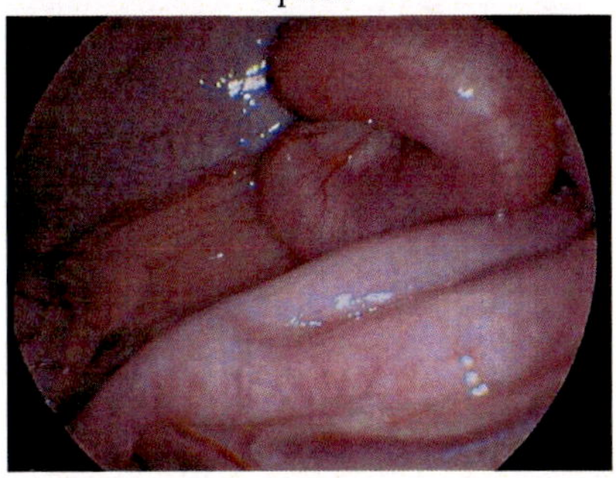

Oviduct

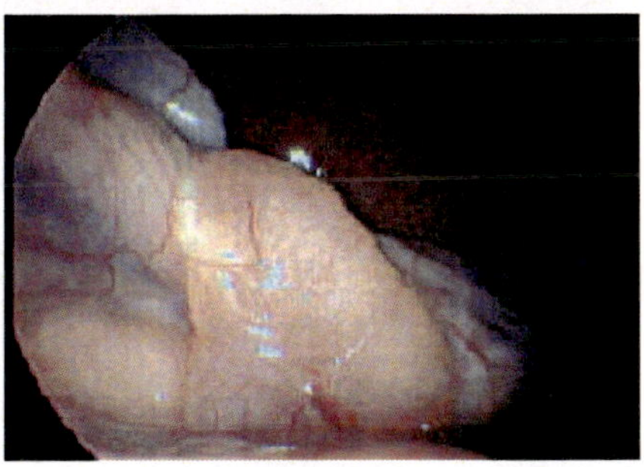

Pancreas

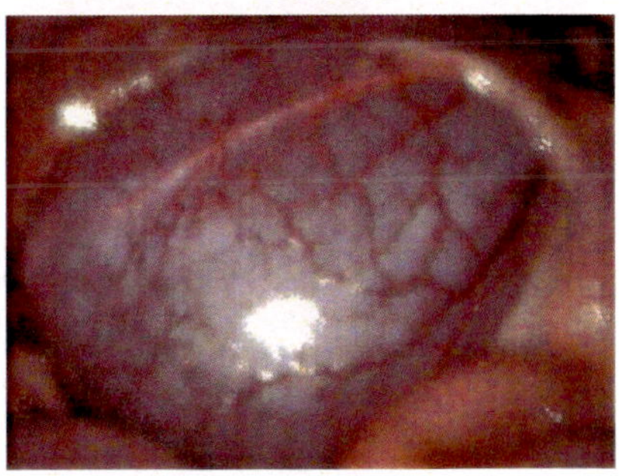

Urinary Bladder

Laparoscopic Diagnosis of different Intraperitoneal lesions

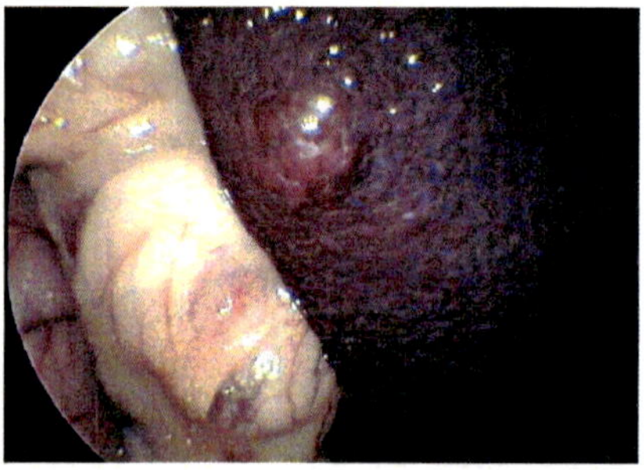

Splenic abscess

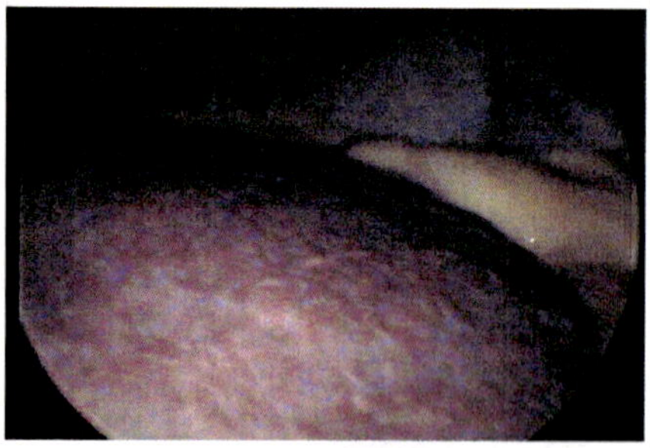

Spleenomegaly

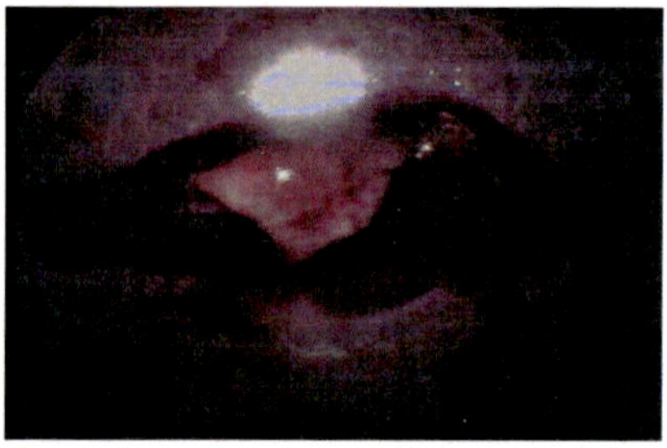

Splenic wound

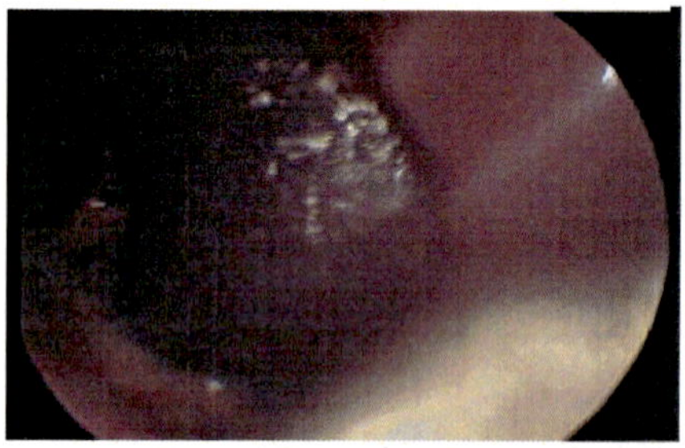

Splenic tumour

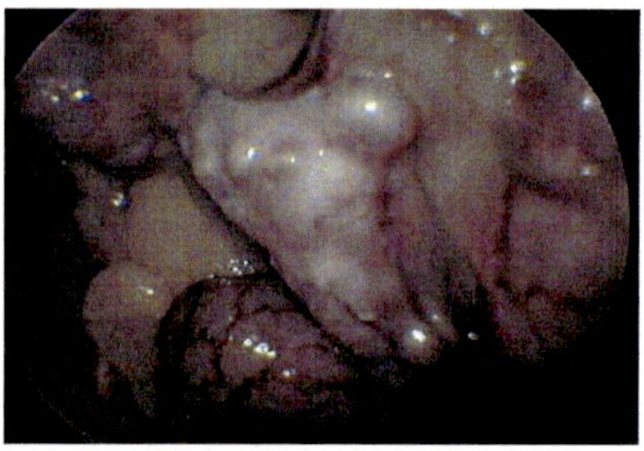

Polycystic ovary

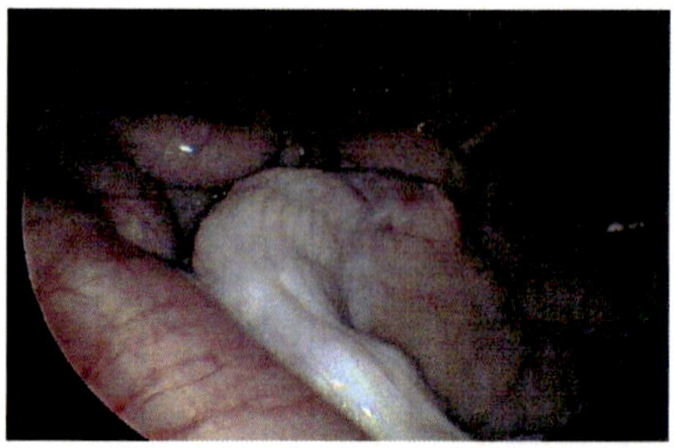

Mummified fetus

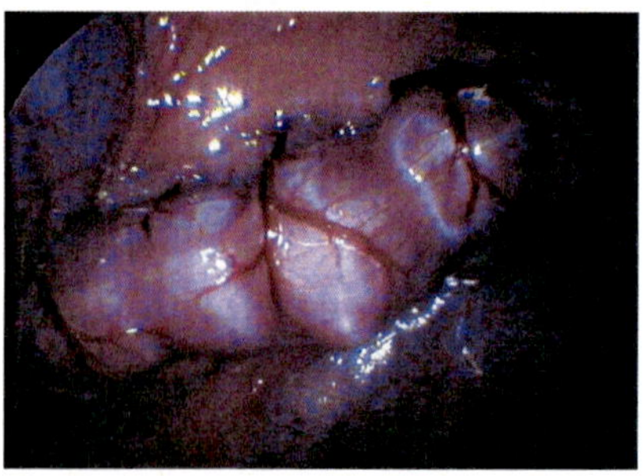

Faecolith

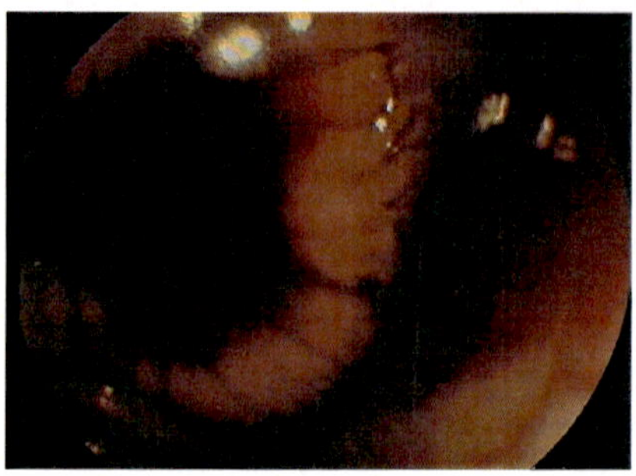

Haemoperitoneum

Laparoscopic diagnosis of intestinal intussusception in dog

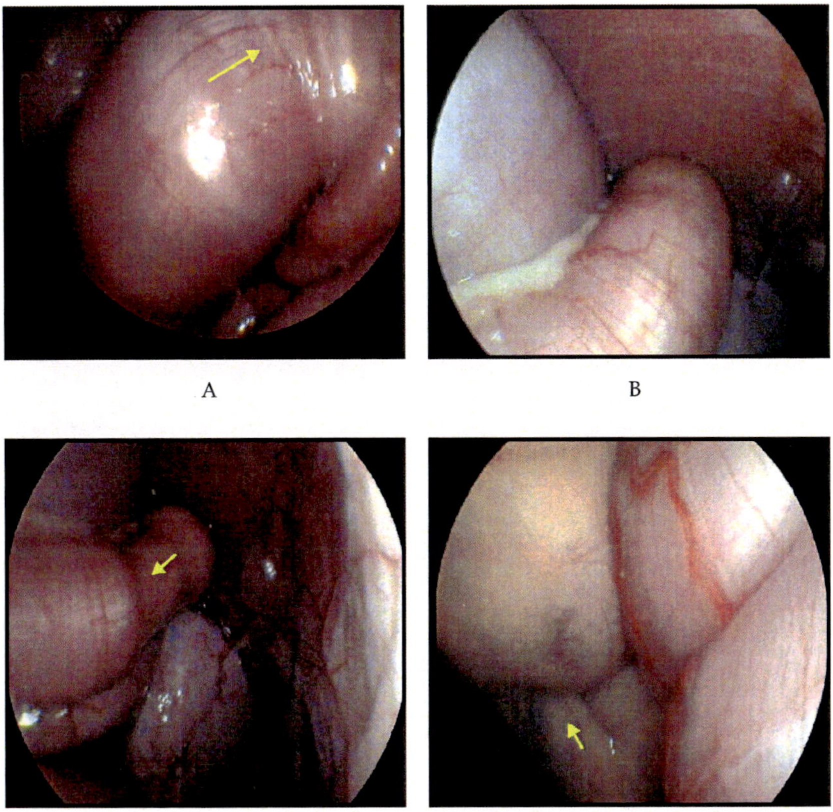

A B C D

Four cases of intestinal intussusception

Chapter 7: Laparoscopic Guided Organ Biopsy and Minor Surgery

Laparoscopic liver biopsy through cauterization in small animal

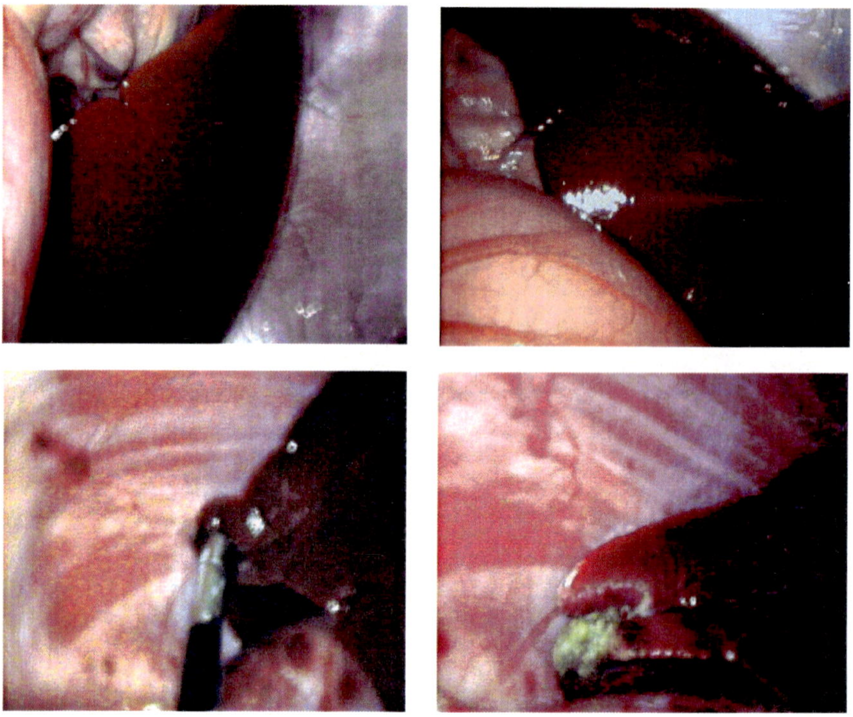

Dog

Laparoscopic liver biopsy through cauterization in small animal

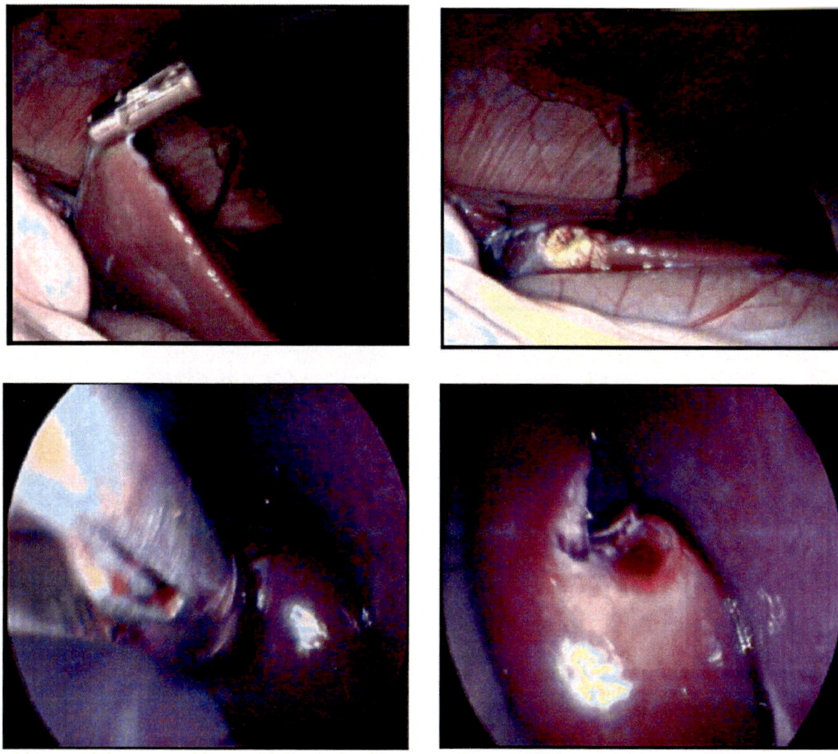

Goat

Laparoscopic liver biopsy through cauterization in small animal

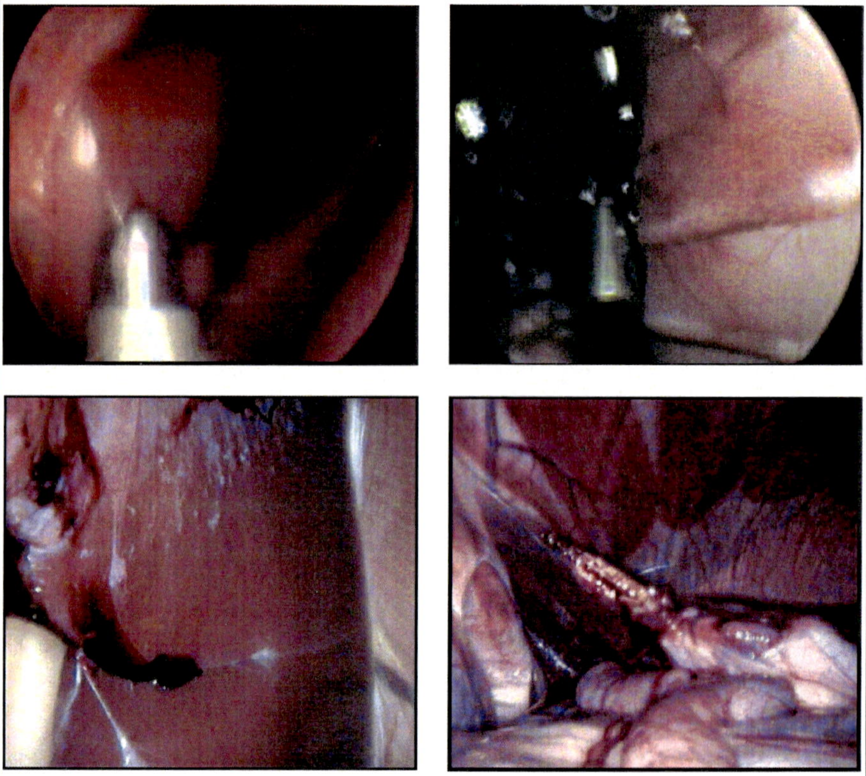

Rabbit

Laparoscopic biopsy of liver and gall bladder

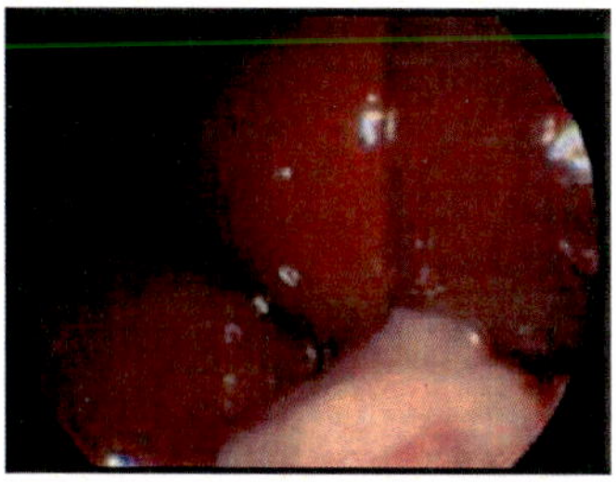

Laparoscopic visualization of liver surface

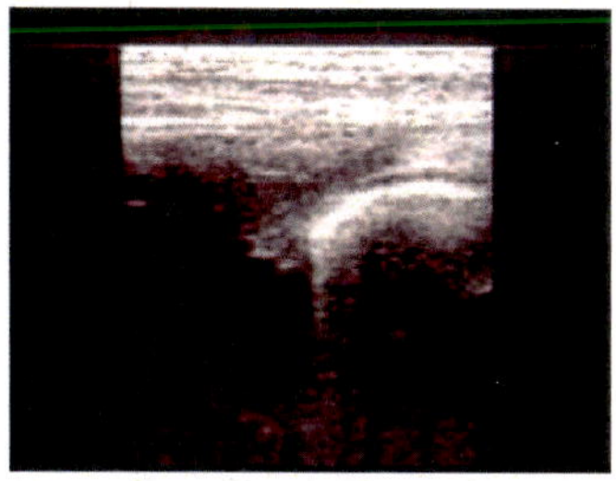

Visualization of liver by ultrasonography

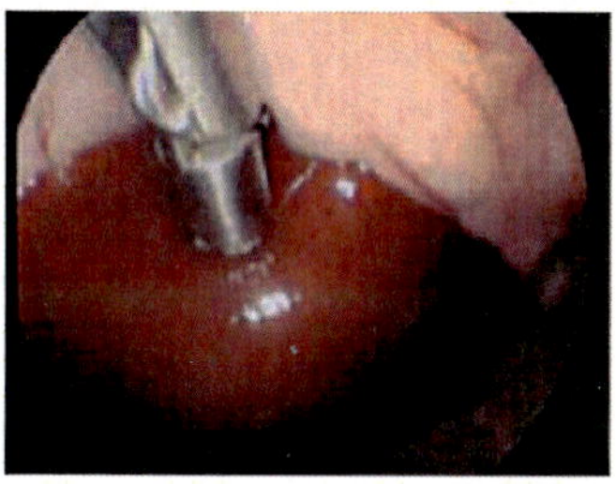

Liver biopsy using biopsy forceps under laparoscopic guidance

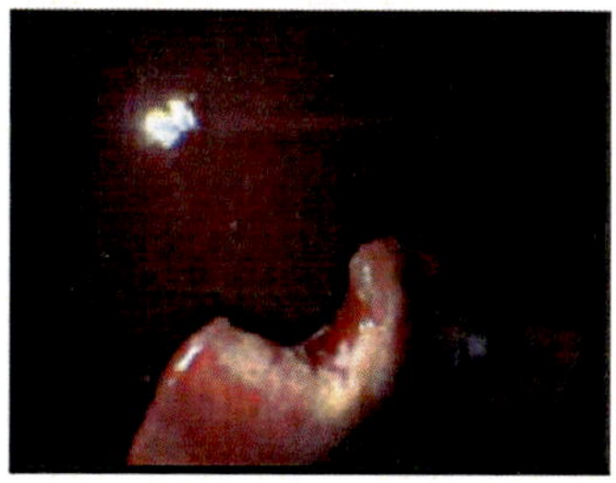

Biopsy site just after laparoscopic biopsy

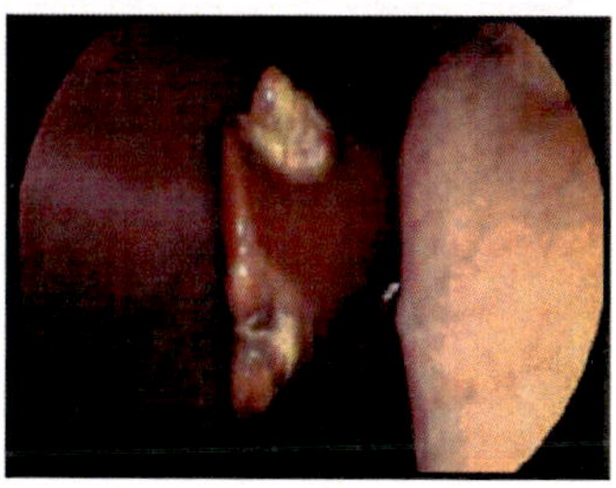

Biopsy site after 7 days of laparoscopic biopsy

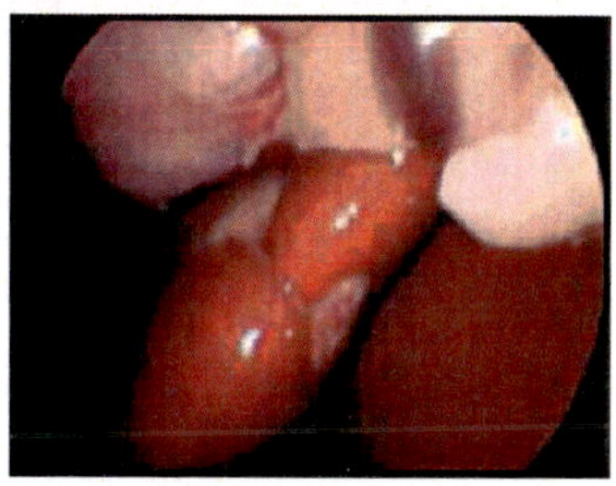

Biopsy site after 15 days of laparoscopic biopsy

Laparoscopic diagnosis of different liver diseases

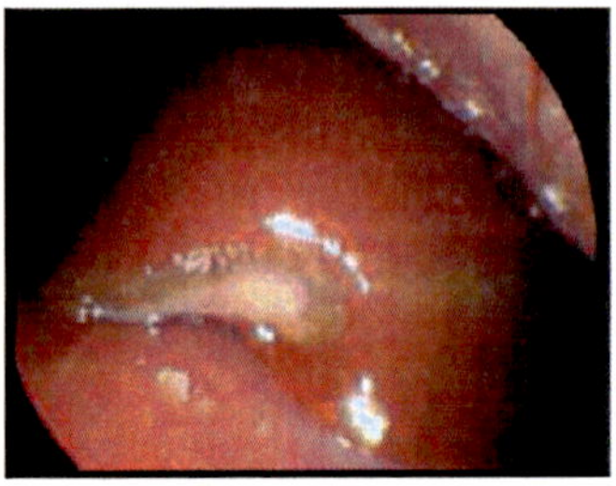

Biopsy site after 30 days of laparoscopic biopsy

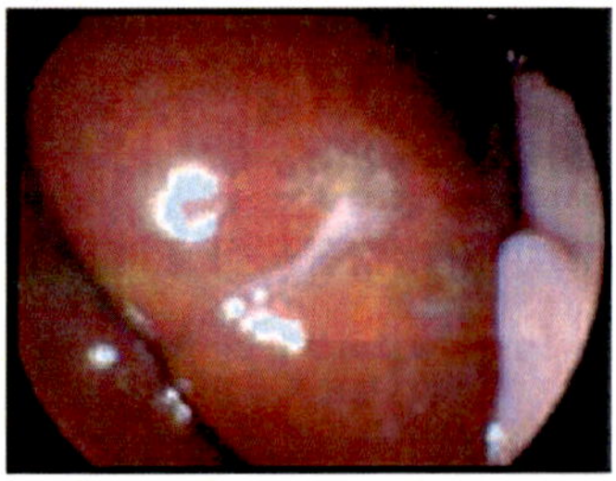

Biopsy site after 60 days of laparoscopic biopsy

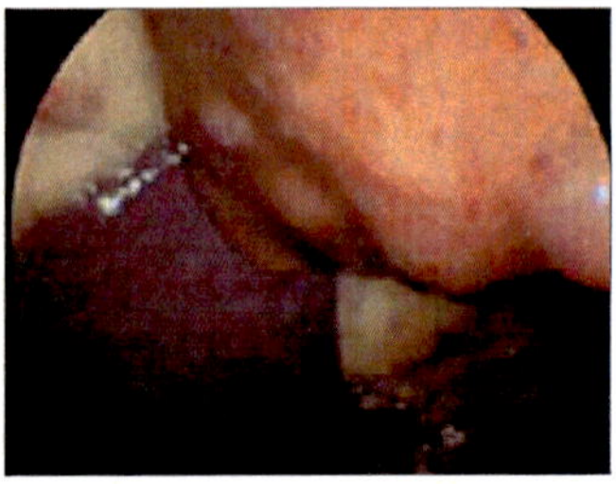

Laparoscopic visualization liposarcoma of liver

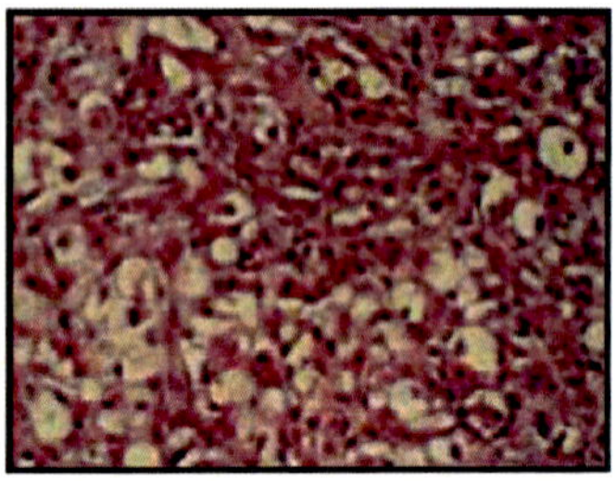

Liposarcoma of liver-tumourous adepocytes lined by hyperchromatic nuclei (H&Ex260)

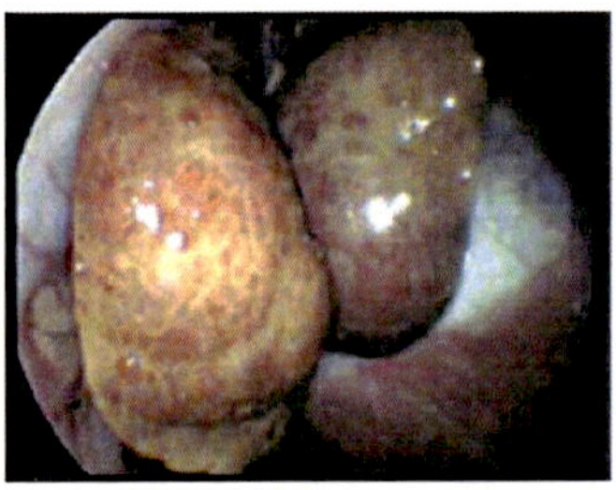

Laparoscopic visualization of liver having cirrhosis

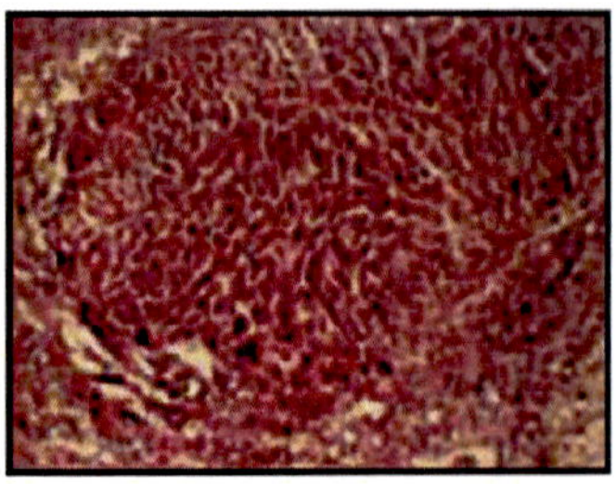

Cirrhosis-hepatocytes surrounded by fibrous connective tissue (H&Ex100)

Laparoscopic diagnosis of different liver diseases

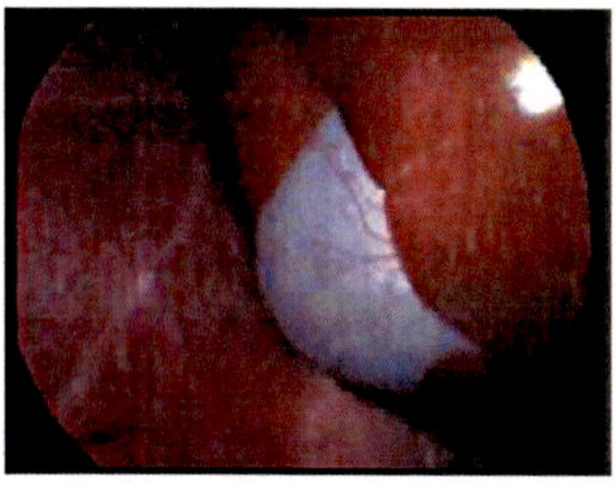

Laparoscopic visualization of hepatitis

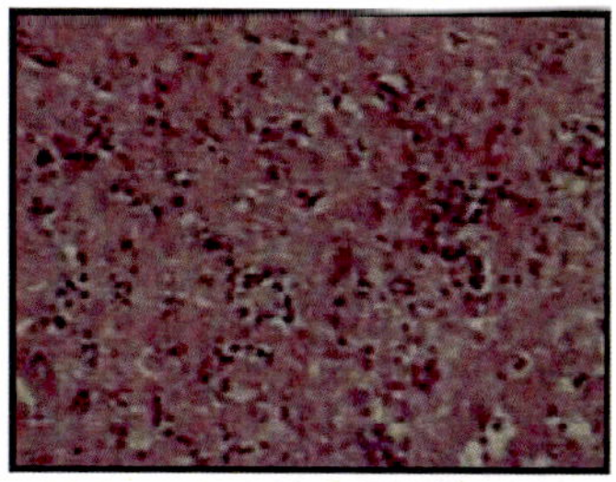

Hepatitis-swollen hepatocytes with large vesicular nuclei and Sinusoids filled with leucocytes (H&E X 260)

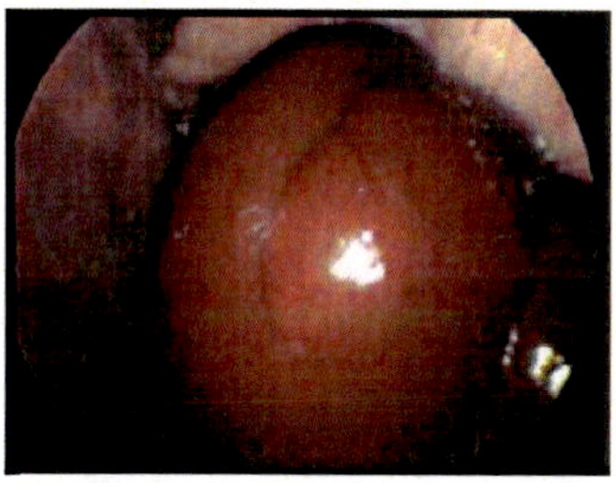

Laparoscopic visualization of hepatomegaly

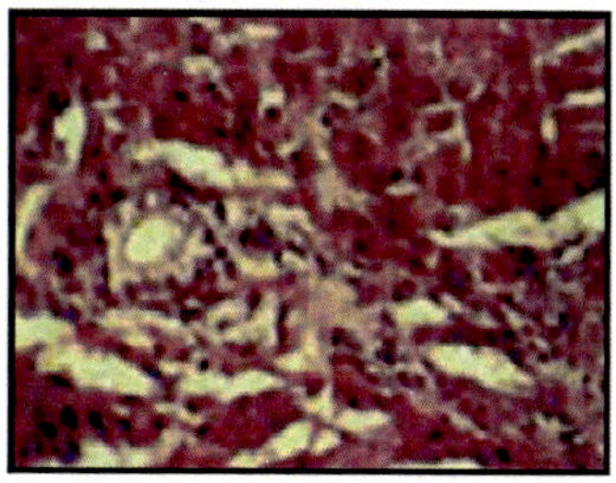

Distended portal area with vacuolated bile duct epithelial cells (H&E X 330)

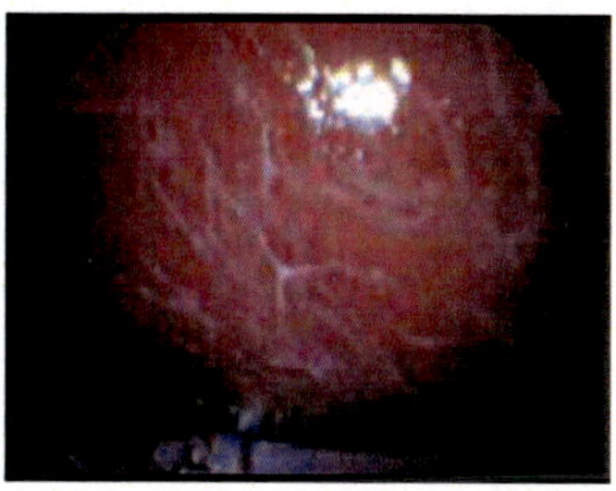

Laparoscopic visualization of liver surface showing bridging fibrosis

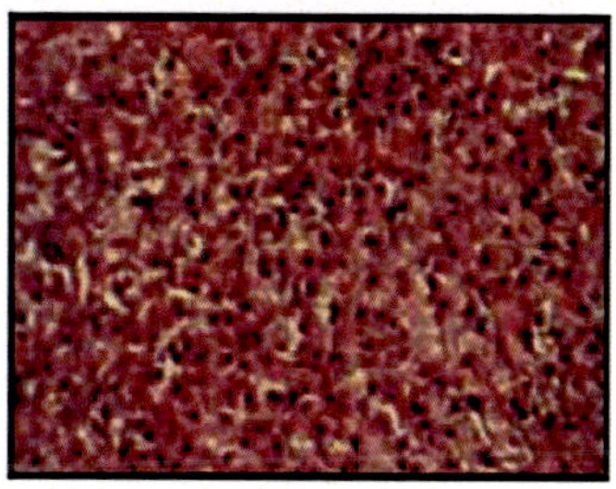

Hepatic parenchyma in dog with bridging fibrosis of liver (H&E X 200)

Chapter 8: Laparoscopic Ancillary Diagnostic Procedures

Instrumentation for laparoscopic biopsy and ancillary procedures

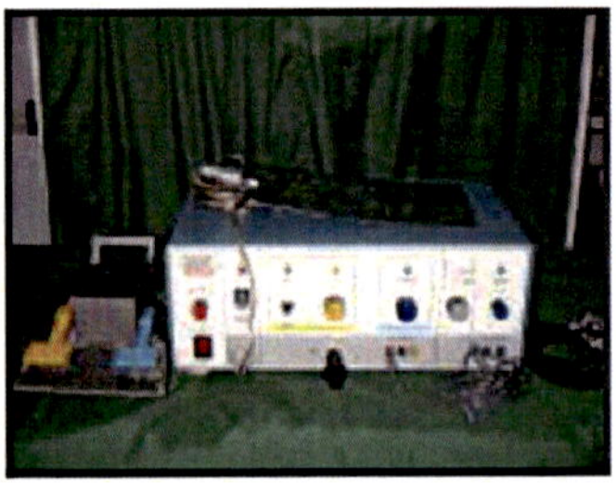

Electro-cautery device
(Megatom 400)

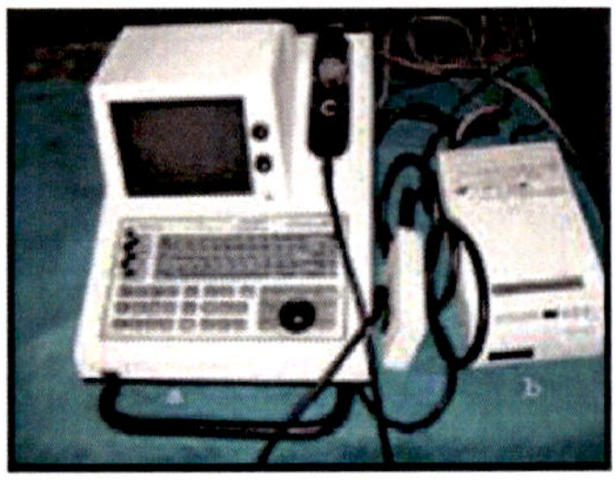

Ultrasonography equipment
a) Monitor, b) Thermoprinter
c) Transducer

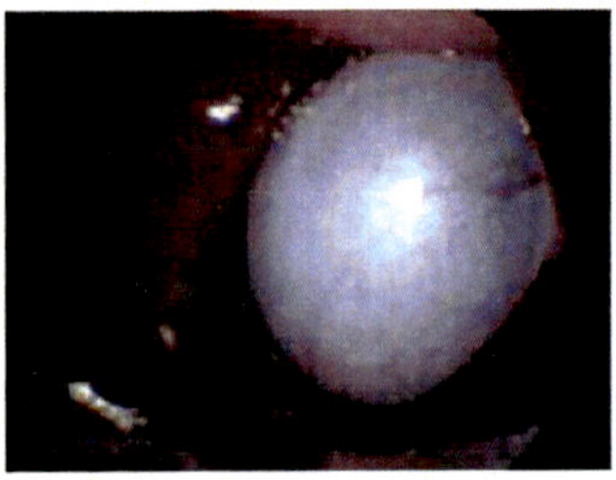

Laparoscopic visualization of gall bladder

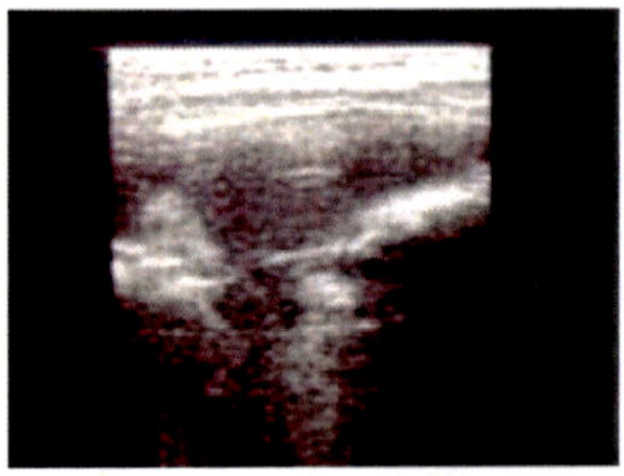

Liver biopsy using percutaneous biopsy needle under ultrasound guidance

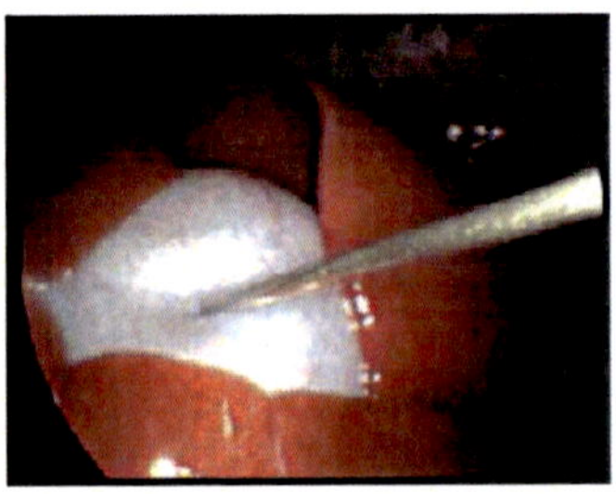

Insertion of spinal needle into gall bladder under laparoscopic guidance

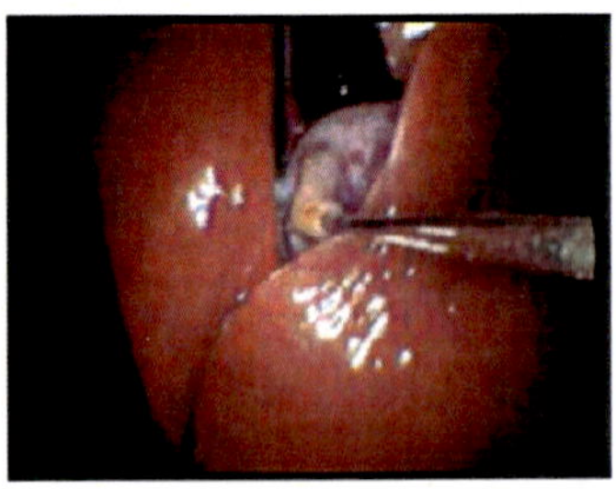

Decompression of gall bladder after aspiration of bile

Laparoscopic guided cholecystography

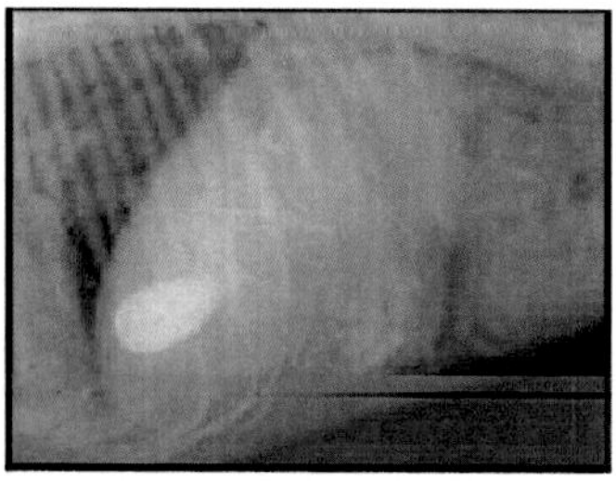

Radiograph taken just after laparoscopy-guided injection of iohexol into Gall bladder

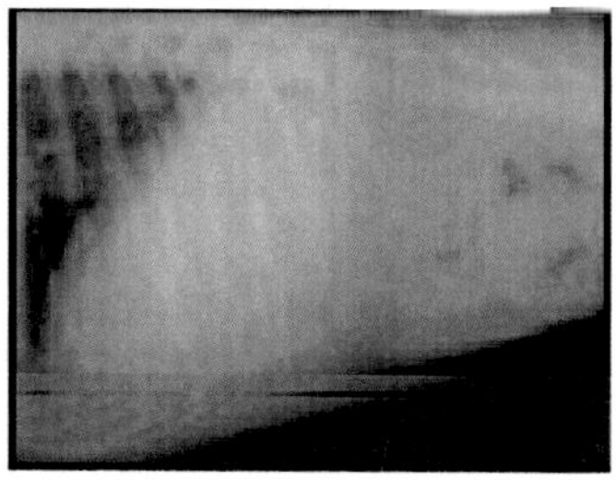

Radiograph taken after 6 hours of a fatty diet following laparoscopic guided Cholecystography

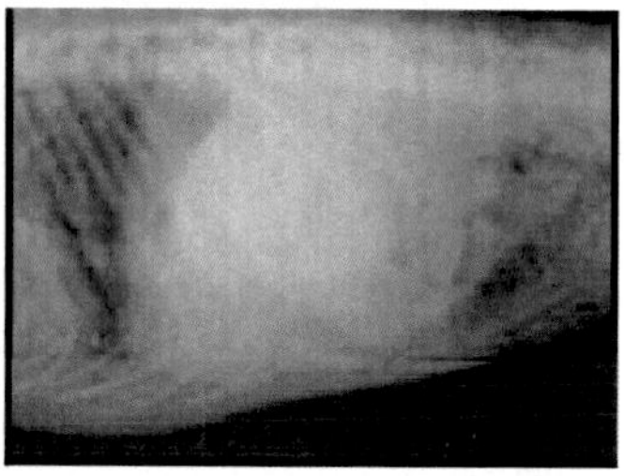

Radiograph taken just after intravenous Cholecystography

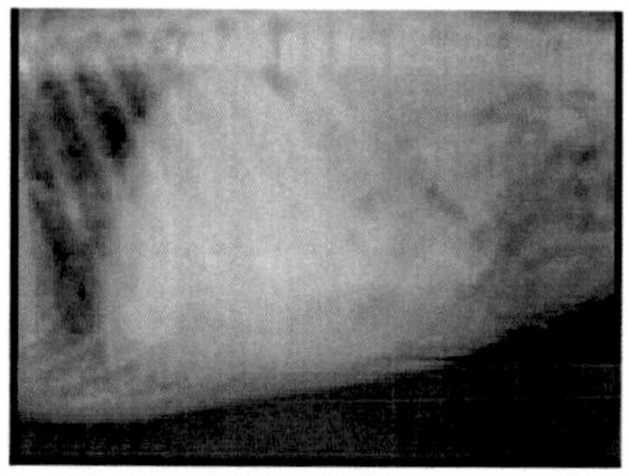

Radiograph taken after 3 hours of intravenous Cholecystography

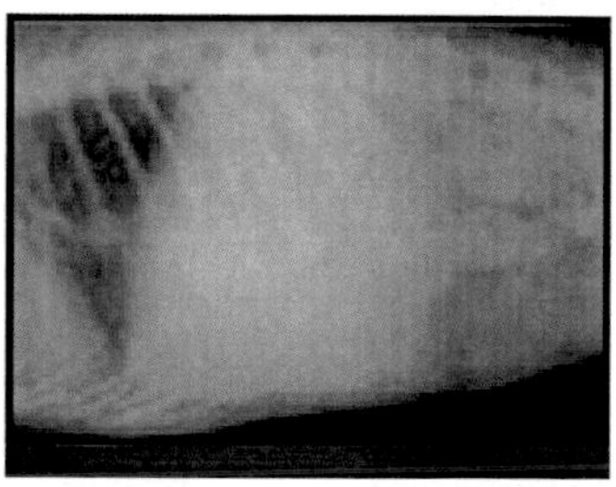

Radiograph taken after 6 hours of a fatty diet following intravenous Cholecystography

Instrumentation for laparoscopic biopsy and ancillary procedures

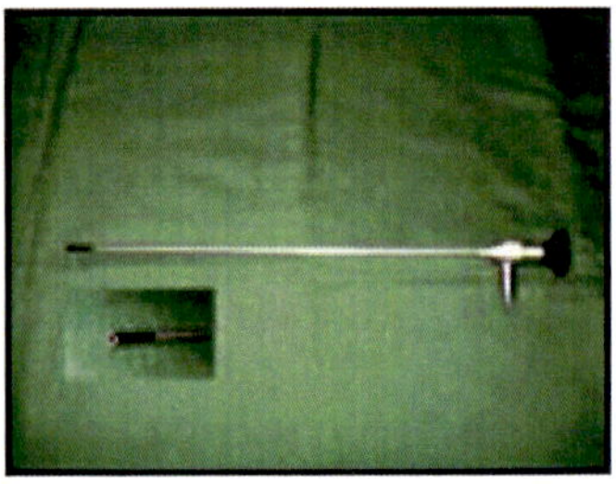

5 mm 30° forward-oblique telescope Distal end of telescope (inset)

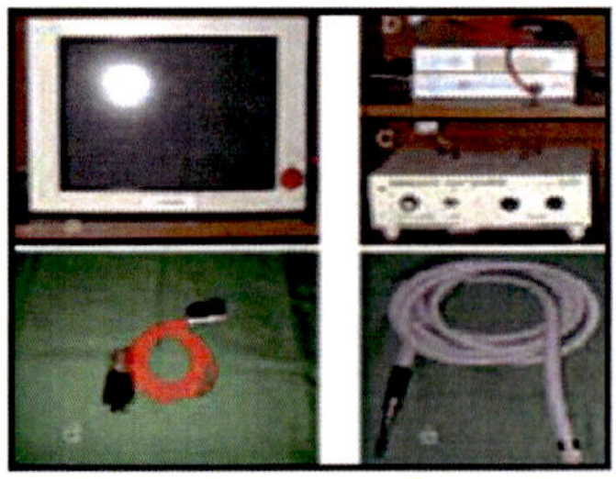

Laparoscopic Image capture system (a) colour monitor (M15E) (b) Image capture device (L-cap) (c) Halogen light source, (d) Endocamera,(e) Fibre-optic cable

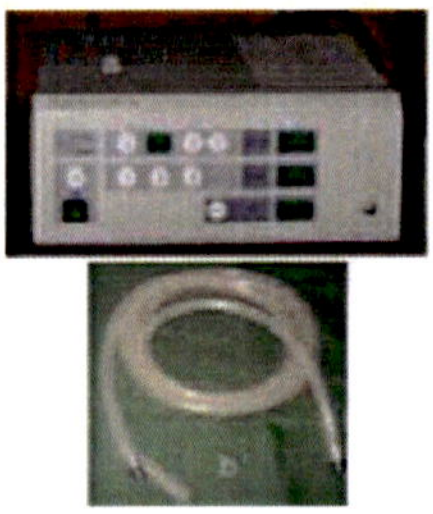

Instruments for abdominal insufflation
a) CO_2 endoflator;
b) CO_2 hose pipe

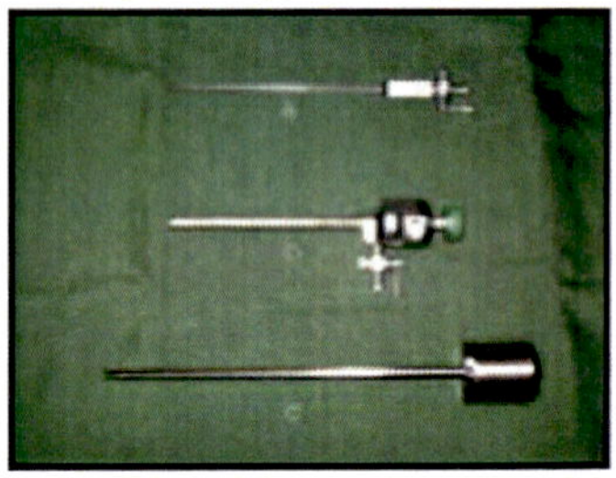

Laparoscopic accessory instruments
a) Veress pneumoperitoneum needle,
b) 5.5 mm cannula
c) Safety trocar

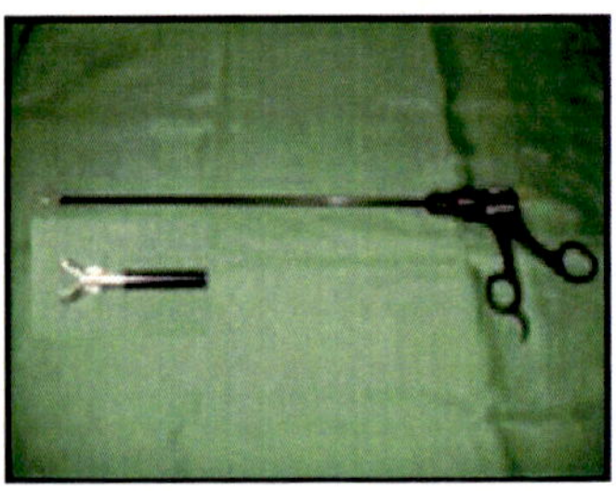

Laparoscopic biopsy forceps
Tip of the forceps (inset)

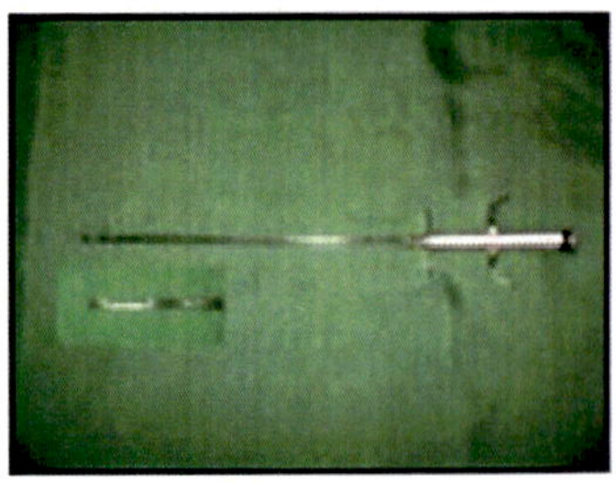

Percutaneous biopsy needle
(Tru-cut type), Tip of the needle (inset)

Chapter 9: Laparoscopic Sterilization in Bitches

Laparoscopic sterilization techniques in bitch (Bilateral oophorectomy)

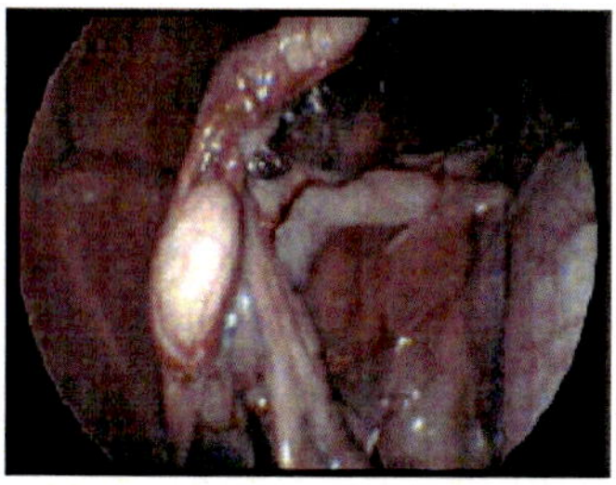

Ovary and mesovarium

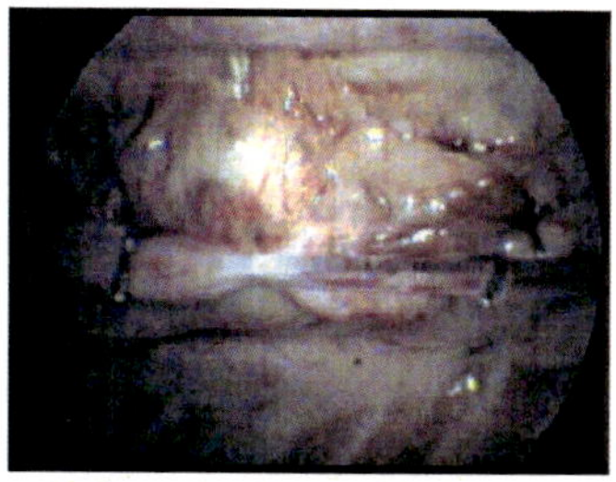

Clip applied both side of the ovary

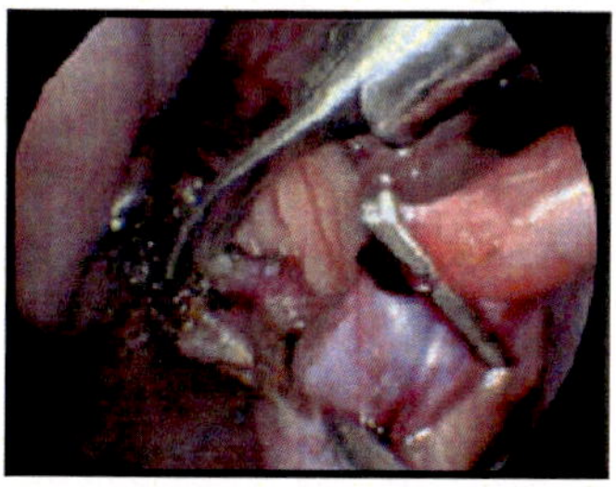

Cauterization and resection of the cranial ovarian attachment

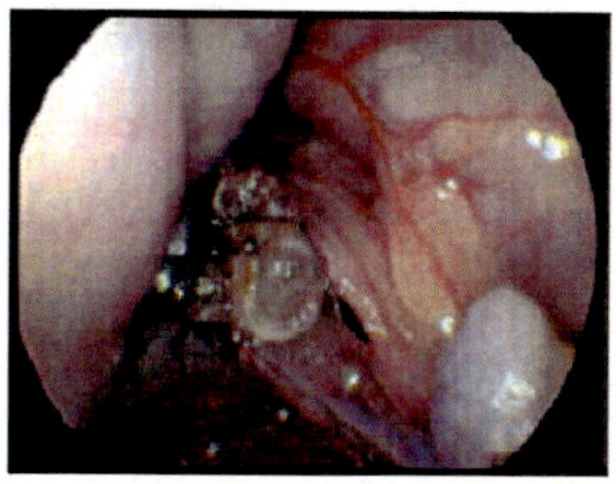

Complete resection of the cranial ovarian attachment

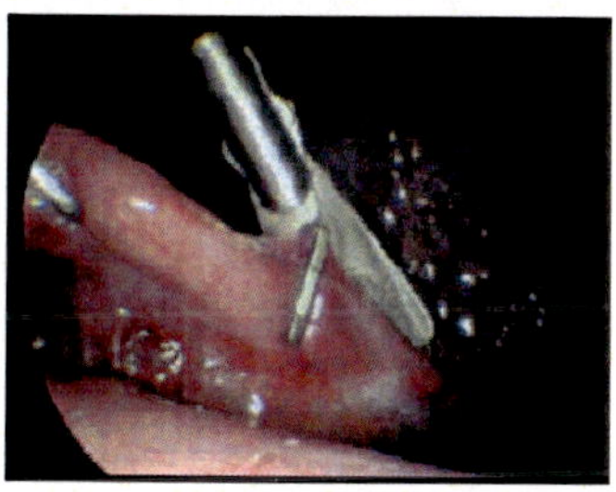

Resection of uterine horn cranial to distal clip

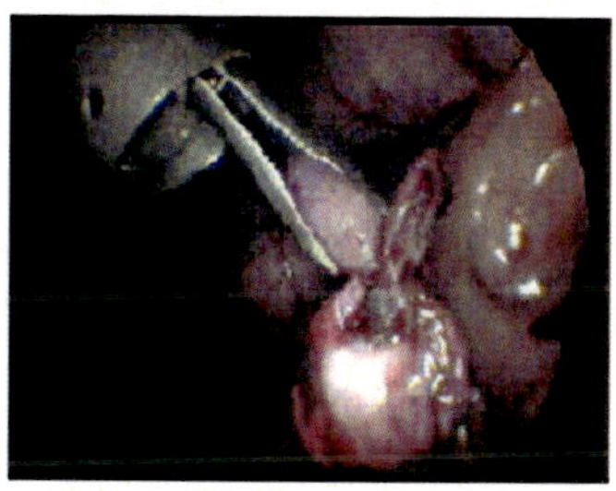

Removal of resected ovary through 10 mm cannula

Laparoscopic sterilization techniques in bitch (Ovariohysterectomy by clip and cautery)

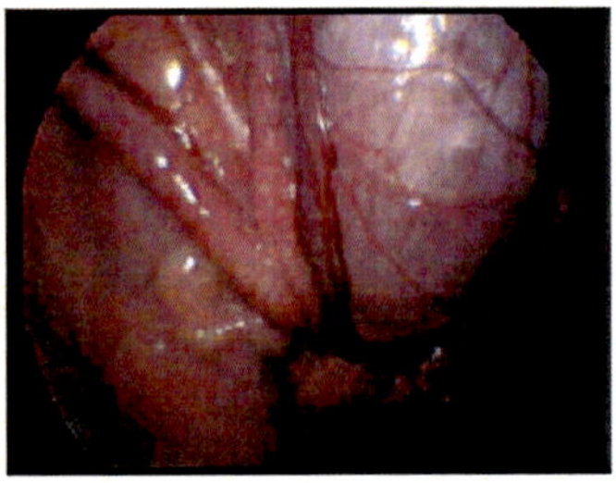

Uterine body and horns

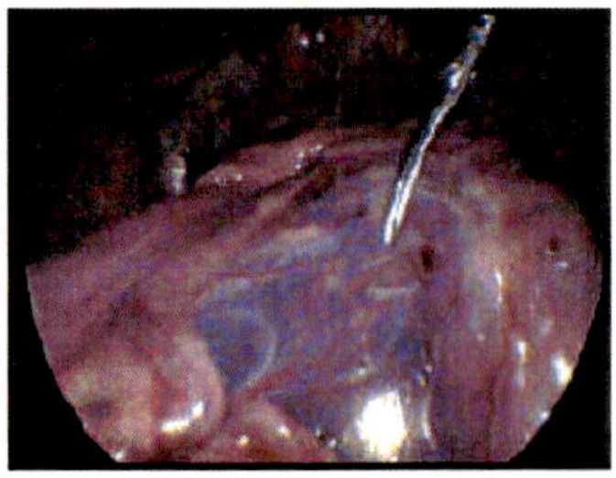

Separation through mesometrium

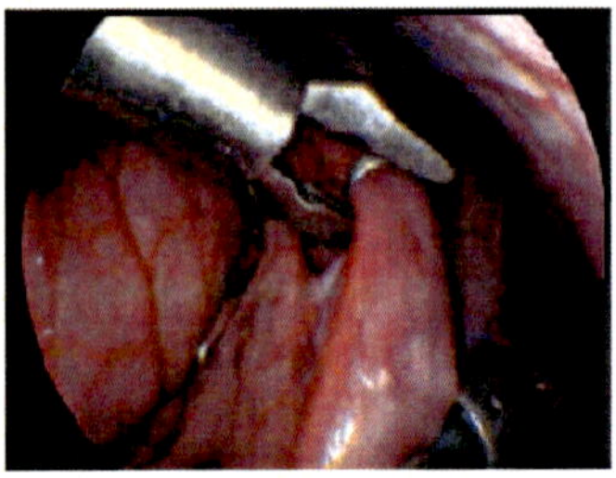

Clipping of uterine body, cranial to cervix

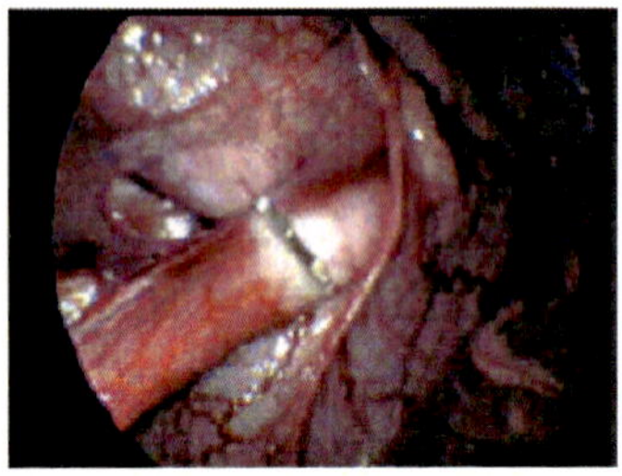

Clipping of uterine body, cranial to cervix

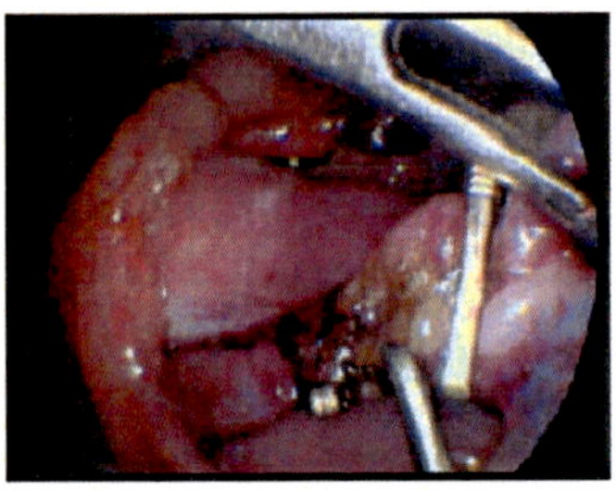

Resection and cauterization of the uterine body after clipping

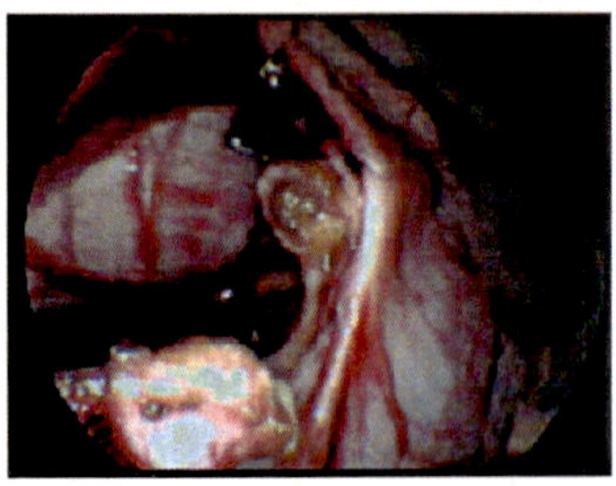

Complete resection of uterine body

Laparoscopic sterilization techniques in bitch (Ovariohysterectomy by electrocautery)

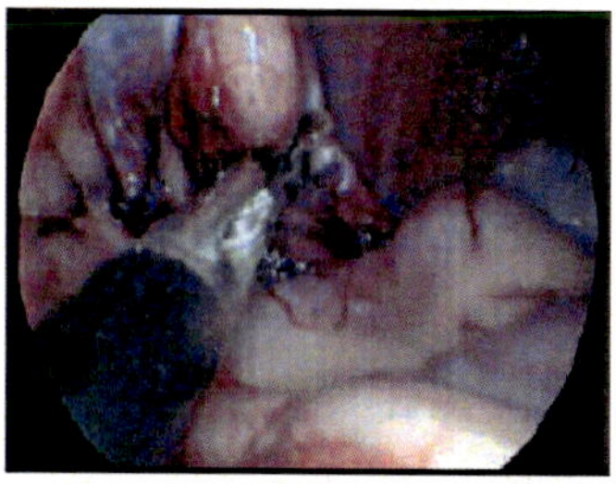

Cauterization and resection of cranial ovarian attachment

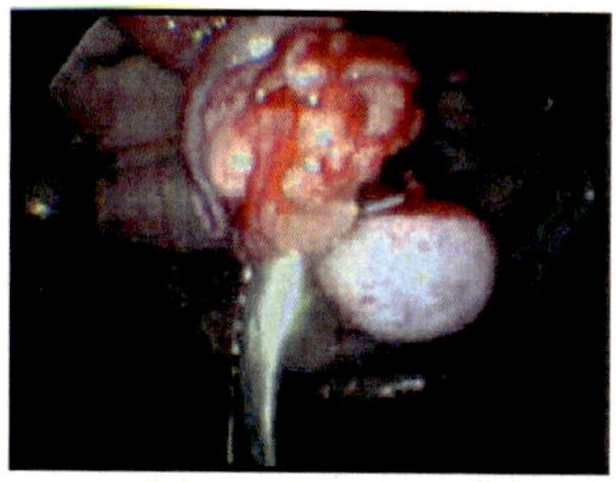

Cauterization and resection of cranial ovarian attachment

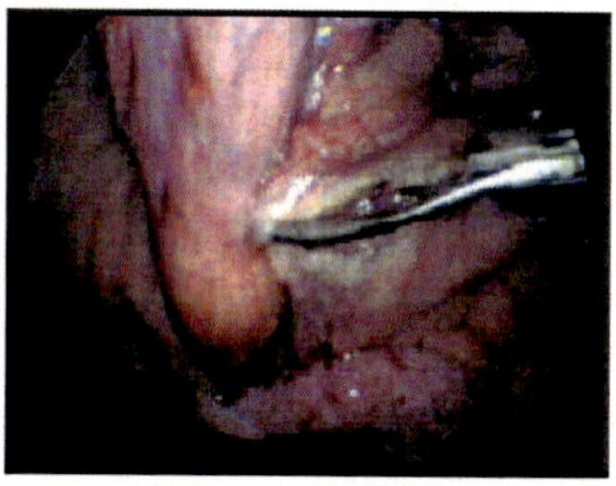

Cauterization and separation of mesometrium

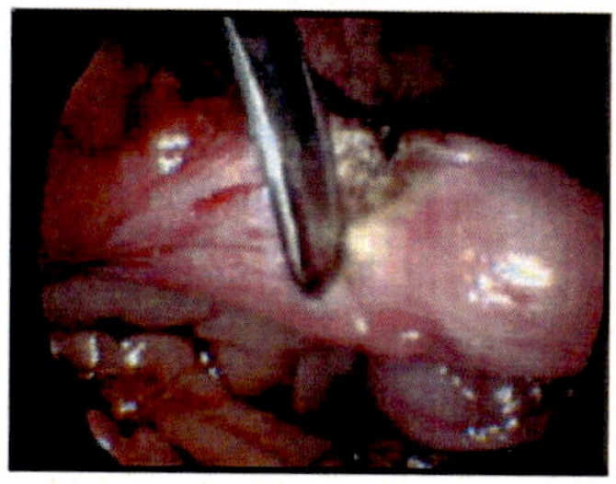

Cauterization and resection of the uterine body

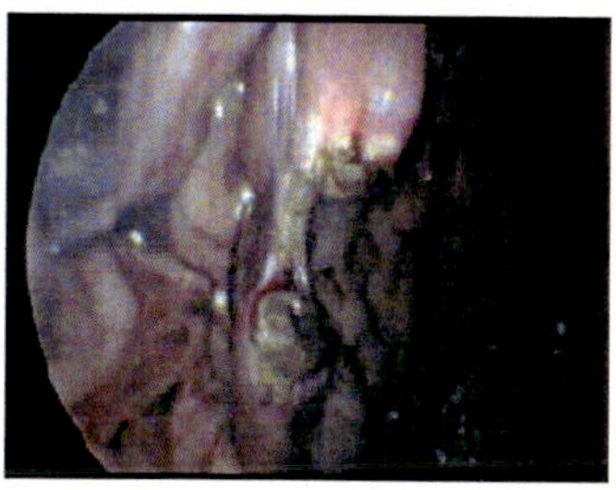

Complete separation of uterine body

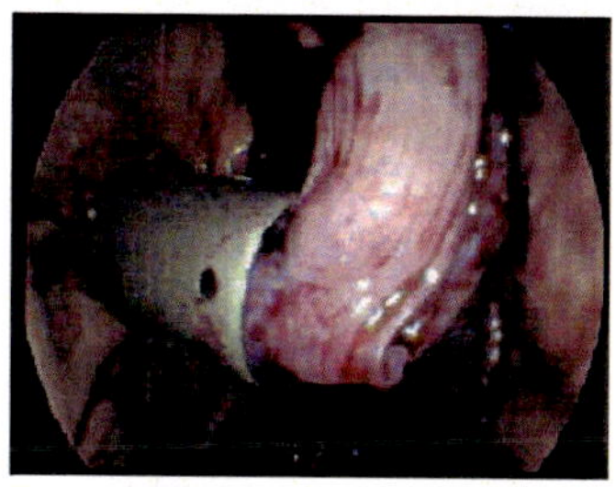

Removal of resected utero-ovarian structure through 10 mm cannula

Chapter 10: Laparoscopic Sterilization in Male Dogs

Laparoscopic sterilization techniques in dogs (Vasectomy)

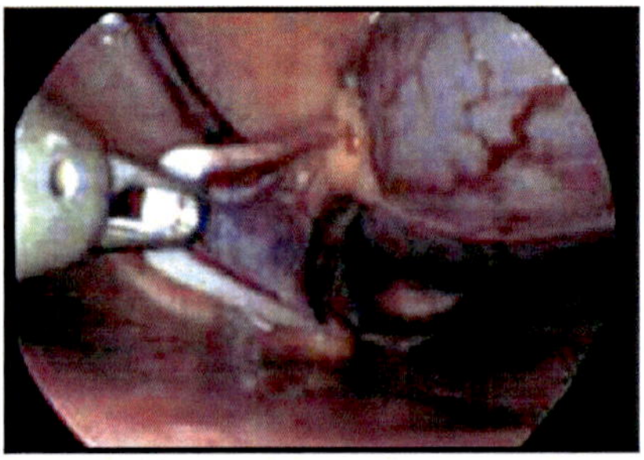

Holding the vas deferens by fenestered grasping forceps for cauterization

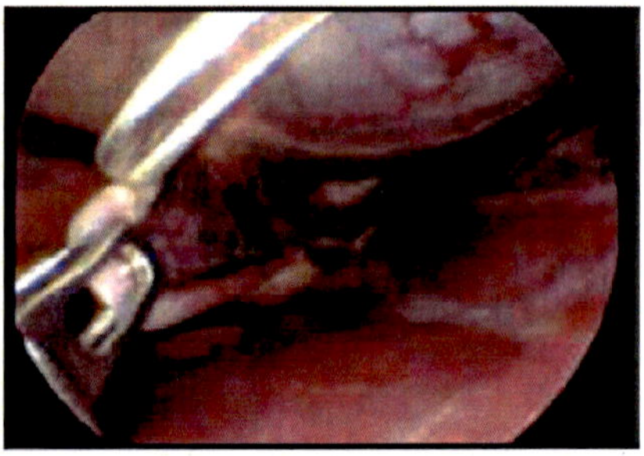

Cauterization of vas deferens by monopolar scissors

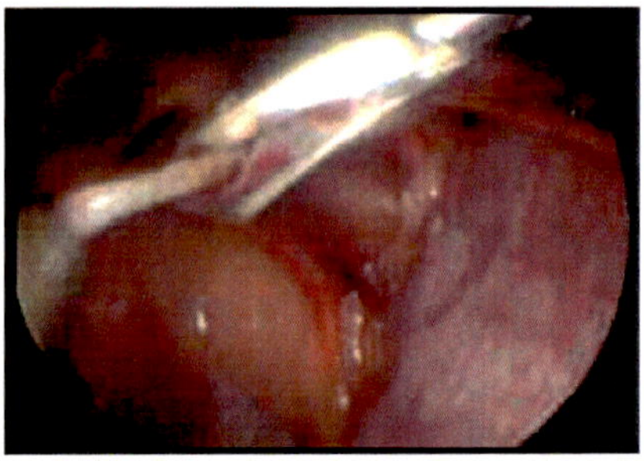

Cutting of vas deferens

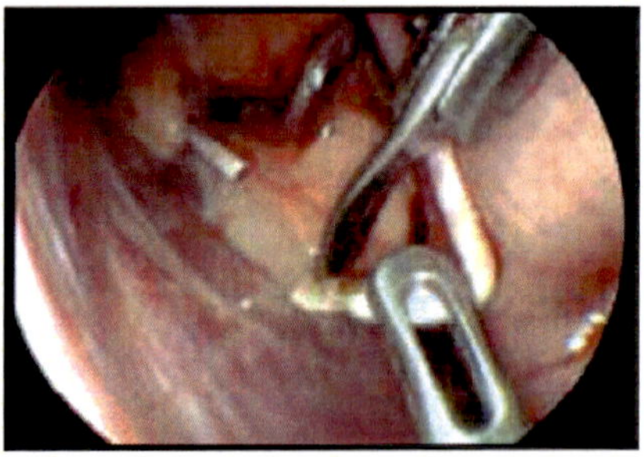

Resection of vas deferens

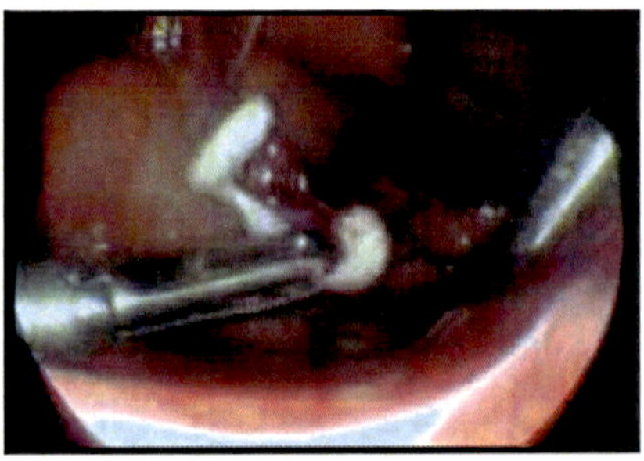

Removal of resected piece of vas-deferens through cannula

NIPA Publications on Veterinary and Animal Husbandry

S.No.	Title	Author	ISBN	Year
1	Analytical Techniques in Animal Nutrition Research	Prabhu, T.M.	9789381450505	2013
2	Animal Breeding and Genetics (As Per VCI Syllabus)	Singh, C.V.	9789383305490	2015
3	Animal Cell Culture and Virology	Nandi, S.	9789380235059	2009
4	Animal Feed Additives	Singh, Pankaj	9789385516092	2015
5	Animal Welfare and Management	BHM Patel, Prasanna, S.B.	9788193014462	2015
6	Applied Veterinary Andrology and Frozen Semen Technology	Shukla, M.	9789380235646	2011
7	Artificial Insemination and Treatment of Infertility in Dairy Animals	Honnappagol, Suresh	9789380235349	2010
8	Avian (Poultry) Production: A Textbook	Sapcota,D.	9789383305476	2014
9	Basics of Research Methodology	Imam,Ekwal	9789383305438	2015
10	Biological Sciences: Innovations and Dynamics	Sinha,Rajeshwar P.	9789383305872	2015
11	Biotechnology in Animal Health and Production	Jindal, S.K.	9789380235356	2010
12	Biotechnology: Practical Manual Series Vol 04	Thara, K.M.	9788190851237	2009
13	Climatic Variability: Impacts on Agriculture and Allied Sectors	Datta, M.:Ed.	9789381450949	2014
14	Clinical Veterinary Medicine: Practical Manual Series Vol 03	Sharma, Neelash	9788190851251	2009
15	Common Reproductive Problems in Bovines and Canines	K.Harendra & Nandi S.	9789380235790	2011
16	Community Ecology of Tropical Birds	Sivaperruman,C. & E.A.Jayson	9789380235165	2010
17	Computers in Agriculture: Fundamentals and Applications	Sharma Manish & Anil Bhatt	9789385516160	2015
18	Dairy Animal Production	Roy,Biswajit	9789383305636	2015
19	Dairy Plant Management	Puranik,D.B.	9789381450864	2014
20	Dairy Technology: Set of 2 Vols.	Singh, Shivashraya	9789381450994	2014
21	Dairy Technology: Vol.01: Milk and Milk Processing	Singh, Shivashraya	9789383305087	2014
22	Dairy Technology: Vol.02: Dairy Products and Quality Assurance	Singh, Shivashraya	9789383305094	2014
23	Diagnostic Veterinary Parasitology: An Introduction	Juyal,P.D.	9789381450901	2013
24	Environmental Changes and Natural Disasters	Babar, Md.	9788189422752	2007
25	Essentials of Toxicology	Matham, Vijay	9789380235783	2011
26	Essentials of Veterinary Diagnostic Imaging	Md.M.Ansari	9789383305148	2014
27	Experimental Biotechnology: Practical Manual Series 06	Dutta, Sunita & Abhijit Dutta	9789380235721	2011
28	Experimental Phytochemical Techniques	Raaman, N.	9789380235943	2012
29	Extension Education Management in Veterinary Sciences and Animal Husbandry	Singh, Ruchi	9789385516054	2016
30	Extension Techniques for Livestock Development	Singh S.K. & S.D.Singh	9789380235233	2011
31	Farm Animal Management: Principles and Practices	Singh, Rana Ranjit	9789383305032	2014

S.No.	Title	Author	ISBN	Year
32	Farm Women Empowerment Through Dairy Co-operative Societies	Swain, Pitambar	9789383305186	2014
33	Forage Conservation Techniques	Pankaj K. Singh	9789383305100	2014
34	Functional Foods	Mishra, H.N.	9789383305988	2016
35	Functional Foods and Nutraceuticals	C.S. Riar, & Saxena,	9789383305964	2015
36	Fundamentals of Veterinary Developmental Anatomy	Rao, Chandrasekhara	9789381450697	2013
37	General Animal Surgery and Anaesthesiology: (With Theory and Practicals)	Gangwar, A.K. Naveen Kumar et.al.	9789380235172	2010
38	Genetic Improvement of Livestock and Poultry	Singh, C.V.& R.S.Barwhal: Ed.	9789381450826	2013
39	Geographic Information System	Gurugnanam, B.	9788190851282	2009
40	Geospatial Technologies for Natural Resources Mgt.	Soam,S.K. & P.D. Sreekant	9789381450802	2013
41	GIS: Fundamentals,Applications and Implementations	Elangovan, K.	9788189422165	2006
42	Glossary of Veterinary Economics	Kumar, Sanjay	9789380235622	2011
43	Goat Production and Health Management	Jindal, S.K.	9789381450536	2013
44	Handbook of Genetics and Biotechnology: Revised and Expanded 2nd ed.	Tomar, R.S.	9789383305445	2014
45	Handbook of Rabbit Production and Management	Rajeshwari, Y.B.	9789380235684	2011
46	Handbook on Care and Management of Laboratory and Pet Animals	Rajeshwari, Y.B.	9788189422981	2009
47	Immunology	Dushyant	9789383305667	2015
48	Immunology of Animal Reproduction	Babu Y.Hari	9789381450727	2013
49	Immunology: At A Glance	Nandi, S.	9788190851213	2009
50	Infectious Diseases of Animals Their Identification and Treatment	Nandi, S.	9789381450390	2012
51	Information Technology in Veterinary Science	Patil, Vivek	9788190851244	2009
52	Introduction to Animal Physiology	Jindal, S.K.	9789380235332	2011
53	Introductory Microbiology	Balachandar, D. & R.T.Vendan	9788189422783	2007
54	Laboratory Manual of Biochemistry: Methods and Techniques	Sengar, R.S.	9789383305025	2014
55	Laboratory Manual of Microbiology: Practical Manual Series: 05	Roy, A.K.	9789380235189	2010
56	Livestock and Poultry: Conservation and Improvement Techniques	Singh, C.V.	9789383305346	2015
57	Livestock Economics: Marketing,Business Management and Accountancy	Gangadhar, K.S.	9788190723701	2009
58	Livestock Entrepreneurship Management	Thakur,Devesh & Pranav Kumar	9789383305650	2015
59	Livestock Nutrition: Analytical Techniques	Gopal Krishna	9789380235967	2012
60	Livestock Production and Management: Recent Trends and Future Prospects	Sunil Kumar: Ed.	9789381450703	2013
61	Mastitis and Allied Diseases in Livestock	De, Ujjwal Kumar	9789381450529	2013
62	Molecular Biology and Biotechnology: Microbial Methods	Parakhia, M.V.	9789380235196	2010
63	Nutraceuticals in Livestock and Poultry	Bhattacharya,Amitav	9789383305674	2015
64	Objective Biochemistry	Sengar,R.S.	9789381450376	2014
65	Objective Genetics	Kumar S. Thirugnana	9789383305605	2015
66	Objective Microbiology	Nandi, S.	9789381450017	2011
67	Practical Animal Nutrition	Mudgal, Vishal	9789380235974	2012

Laparoscopic sterilization techniques in dogs (Vasectomy + clipping of spermatic plexus)

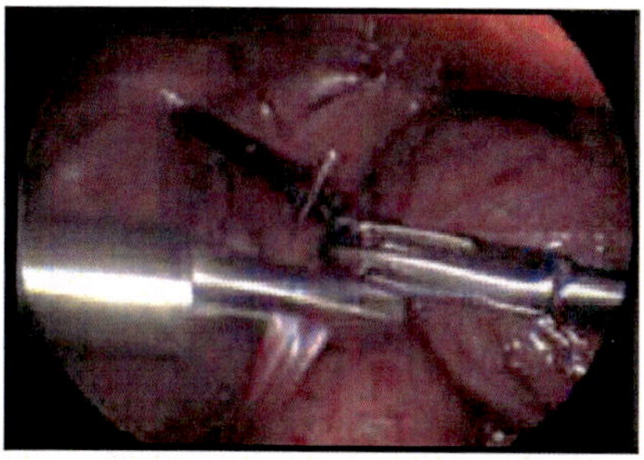

Application of second endoclip in spermatic artery-vein plexus

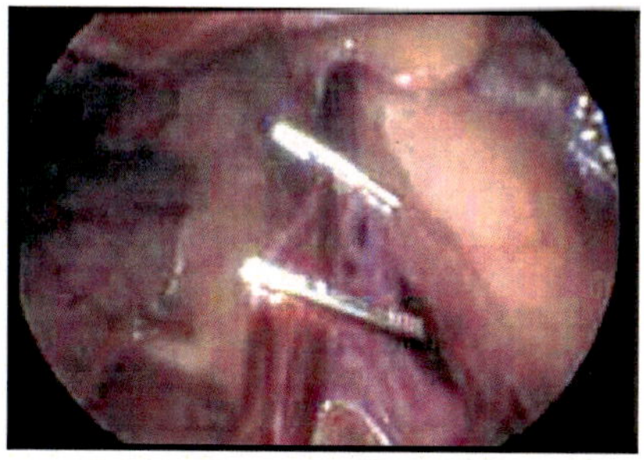

Two endoclips applied to spermatic artery-vein plexus

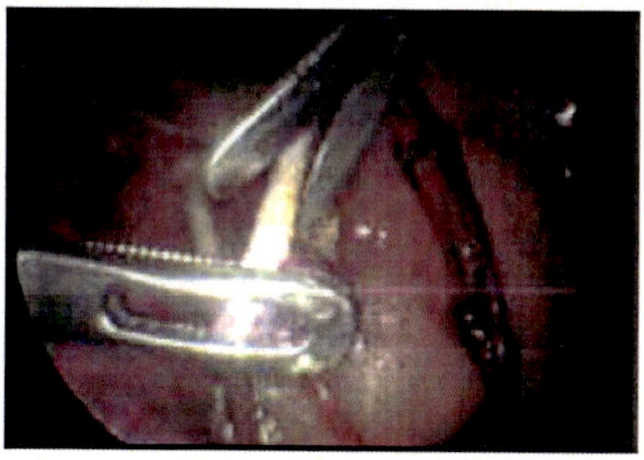

Cauterization and cutting of vas deferens

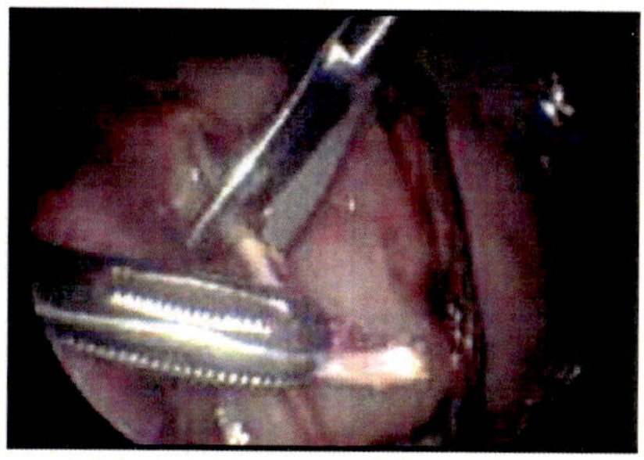

Resection of vas deferens

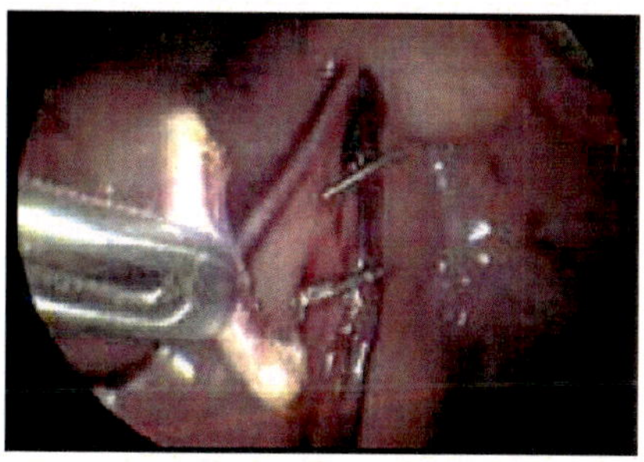

Removal of resected piece of vas deferens outside

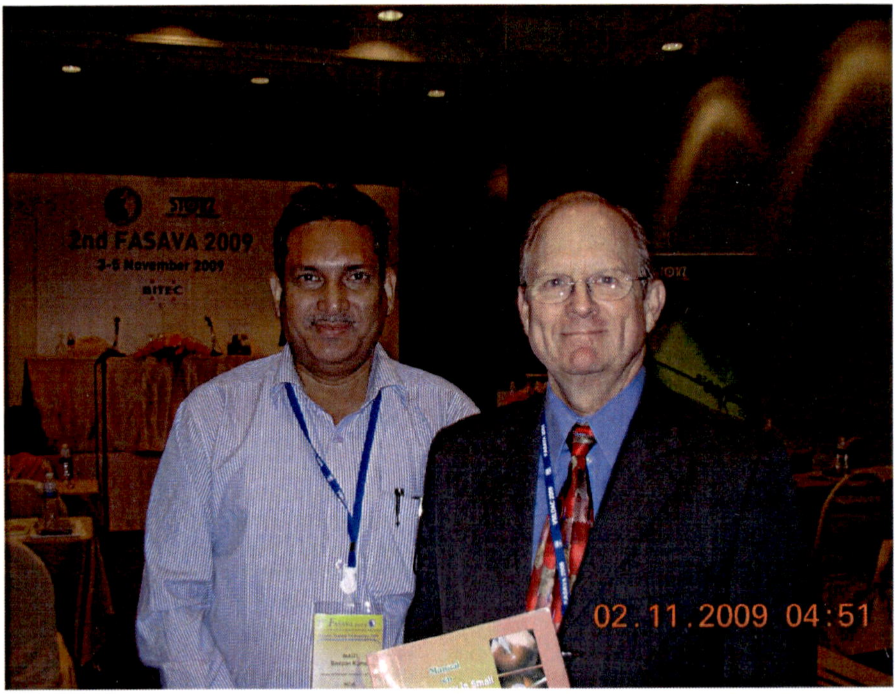

"Our Inspiration"

Prof. (Dr) David C Twedt with Senior Author

Address of Veterinary Laparoscopic Instruments

1. **KARL STORZ Endoscopy India Private Ltd.**
   C-126, Okhla Industrial Area, Phase-1,
   New Delhi-110 020
   Tel: 011-43743000-30, 011-2681 5445-48
   E-mail: corporate@karlstorz.in

2. **Frontline Electro Medical Ltd.**
   Plot No. 9, Local shopping Complex, Surajmal Vihar
   New Delhi-110 092
   Tel: 011-22375294/22375092
   Email: info@feml.in

S.No.	Title	Author	ISBN	Year
68	Principles of Meat Technology: 2nd Revised and Expanded ed.	Singh V.P. & Neelam Sachan	9789383305797	2015
69	Quality Assessment of Milk & Milk Products	Thompkinson, D.K.	9789381450444	2012
70	Quality Assurance Techniques in Pharmaceuticals	Waghulkar, V.M.	9789381450130	2012
71	Quality Milk Production and Processing Technology	Thompkinson, D.K. & Latha Sabikhi	9789380235899	2012
72	Question Bank in Extension Education	Mohammad,Asif	9788193014493	2015
73	Rabbit Production and Management	Bandey, M.T.	9789383305391	2014
74	Recent Trends in Animal Behaviour	Sridhara, Shakuntala	9788189422547	2009
75	Rural Livelihood and Food Security	Wani, M.H.	9789380235936	2012
76	SHGs in Techno-Economic Empowerment of Tribal Women	Satapathy, C. & Sabita Mishra	9789380235875	2011
77	Social-Ecological Diversity and Traditional Food Systems	Singh,Ranjay Nancy J.Turner	9789383305360	2014
78	Swine Production and Health Management	Dimri,U. & M.C. Sharma	9789381450161	2013
79	Technologies for Livelihood Enhancement	V.L. Chopra	9789383305810	2015
80	Textbook of Ruminant Nutrition	Mondal, G.	9789381450062	2012
81	The Qur-anic Plants and Animals	Zeerak, Nazir Ahmad	9789383305780	2015
82	Transgenic Animals in Agriculture: Indian Print	Murray, J.D.	9788189422073	2005
83	Veterinary Bacteriology	Samanta, Indranil	9789381450550	2013
84	Veterinary Epidemiology: Basic Concepts	Rajkumar, K.	9789383305131	2014
85	Veterinary Toxicology	Matham, Vijay	9788190723749	2009
86	Vet's Ready Reckoner	Patri, Sravanthi & Vijay Matham	9788190723732	2009
87	Women in Agriculture and Rural Development	S., Shakuntala: eds.	9788189422998	2009
88	Women in Sustainable Agriculture	C.Satapathy & Sabita Mishra	9789383305056	2014
89	Youth in Agriculture and Rural Development	K.Narayana Gowda:Ed.	9789381450758	2013
90	Zoonotic Diseases	Nandi,S.	9789381450963	2014